Fundamental Strength Training After 50

Simple weight training exercises to maintain health, increase functional fitness, lose fat & improve strength beyond 50. (Simple Fitness After 50: Book One)

Mike Wilson

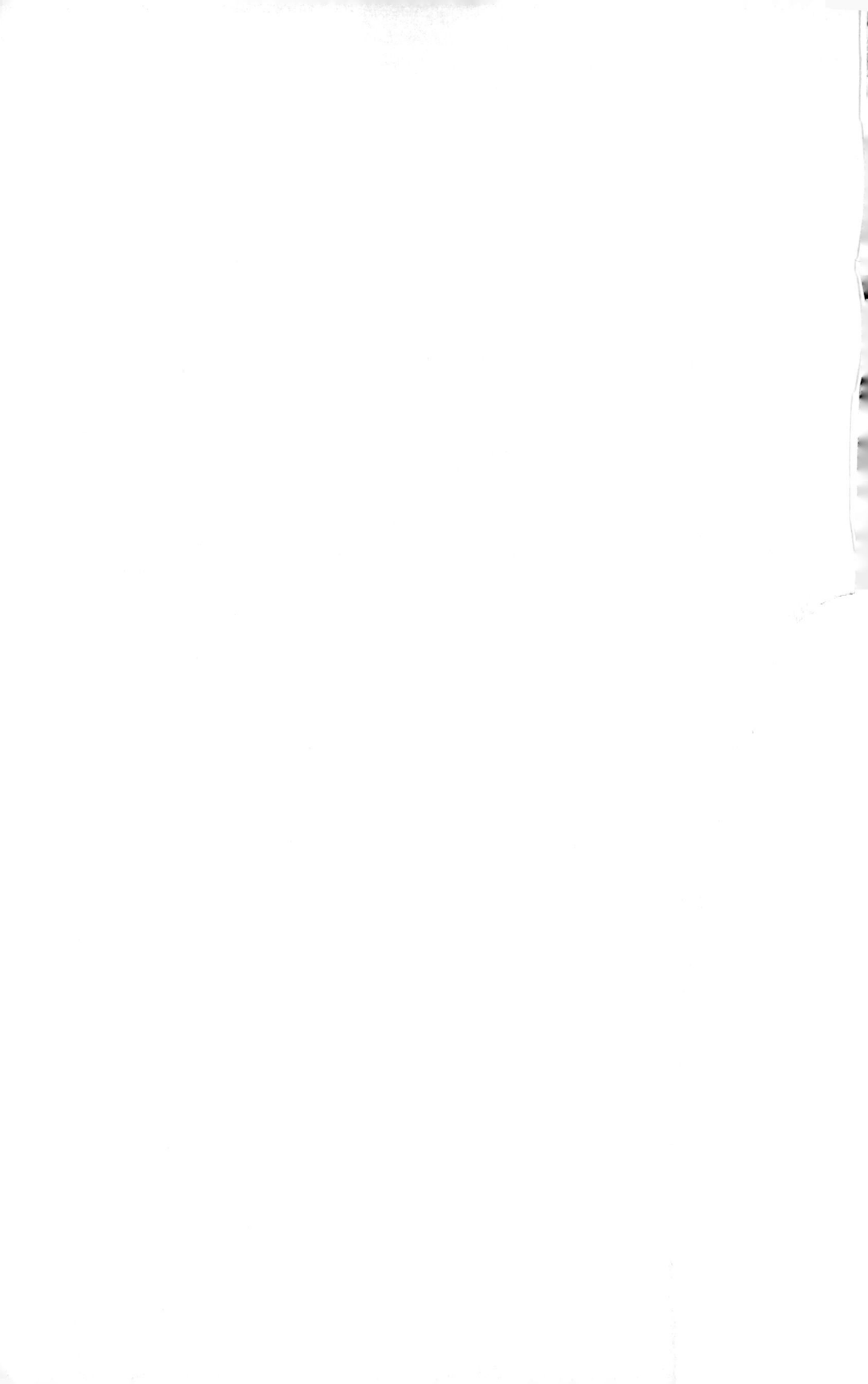

Copyright © 2022 by Mike Wilson.

All rights reserved.

The content contained within this book may not be reproduced, duplicated, distributed or transmitted in any form or by any means, without the direct permission of the author or publisher. You cannot amend, resell, use, quote, or paraphrase any part without written consent from the author or publisher.

Disclaimer

Although the author and publisher have made every effort to ensure that the information in this book was correct at press time, the author and publisher do not assume and hereby disclaim any liability to any party for any loss, damage, or disruption caused by errors or omissions, whether such errors or omissions result from negligence, accident, or any other cause.

The information contained within this book is for educational and entertainment purposes only and should not be used to replace the specialized training and professional judgment of fitness, health care or mental health professionals. All effort has been made to present accurate, up to date, and reliable information. No warranties of any kind are declared or implied. Readers acknowledge the author is not engaging in the rendering of legal, financial, medical or professional advice. The content of this book has been derived from various sources. Please consult a licensed professional before attempting any techniques outlined in this book.

By reading this book, the reader agrees that under no circumstances is the author responsible for any losses, direct or indirect, which are incurred because of the use of the information contained within this book, including, but not limited to; errors, omissions, or inaccuracies. The author is not responsible for any injuries that might occur because of using the exercises recommended in this book. Under no circumstances will any blame or legal responsibility be held against the publisher or author for any damages, reparation, or monetary loss because of the information contained within this book.

You should consult your GP/physician or another health professional before starting this or any other fitness program to determine if it is suitable for your personal needs. This is particularly true if you, or your immediate family, have a history of high blood pressure or heart disease, have ever experienced chest pain when exercising or have experienced chest pain in the past month when not engaged in physical activity. Also, if you smoke, have high cholesterol, are obese, or have a bone or joint problem that could be made worse by a change in physical activity. Do not start this fitness program if your GP/physician or other health professional advises against it. If you experience dizziness, faintness, pain or shortness of breath at any time while exercising, stop immediately and seek professional advice.

Contents

Free Bonus Material   IX
1. The "Simple Fitness After 50" Series   1
2. Introduction   5
3. The Aging Process   9
4. Strength Training Principles   11
   Benefits of Strength Training After 50
   Types of Strength Training
   Home-Based Strength Training Equipment
   Are All Strength Training Exercises 'Good'?
   Compound Exercises vs. Isolation Exercises?
   Training Terminology
5. Habit vs Quick Fix   23
   Outcome vs Process Goals
   SMART Goals
   Short, Medium and Long-term Goals
6. Health Screening   29
   Physical Activity Readiness Questionnaire (PAR-Q)
   Resting Blood Pressure
   Resting Heart Rate

7. Tracking Progress — 35
   Importance of Tracking Progress
   How to Track Progress
   Health & Fitness Tests

8. Myths & Misconceptions — 47
   Common Myths

9. Warm Up and Cool Down — 51
   Warm Up & Dynamic Stretches
   Cool Down & Static Stretches

10. General Exercise Technique — 55
    Spinal Alignment
    Hip-Knee-Ankle (H-K-A) Alignment
    Wrist Alignment
    Range of Motion (ROM)
    Tempo
    Breathing

11. The Essential Eight — 59
    The Squat
    The Hip Hinge
    The Step Up
    The 'Pull'
    The Horizontal Pull
    Vertical Pull
    The 'Push'
    The Horizontal Push
    The Vertical Push
    The Carry
    The Essential Eight Summary

12. 8 Week Program 145
    Terminology Reminder
    Planning
    Progressing
    8 Week Example Programs

13. Conclusion 157

Thank You and Please! 159

Author Bio 161

Coming Soon 163

Bibliography 165

Free Bonus Material

GRAB YOUR FREE BONUS MATERIAL NOW!

I've tried to pack as much information into this book as possible. However, I want you to have access to even more content that cannot be put into book format.

To make sure you get as much value as possible from this book, I've put together FREE additional content for you, including:

- Videos demonstrating the technique for all exercises within this book, plus additional variations of those exercises.
- A video demonstrating a comprehensive Warm Up to prepare for the strength training exercises.
- A video demonstrating Cool Down Stretches to be performed after the strength training exercises.
- A printable PDF version, including exercise illustrations, of the 8 week strength training program.
- A regular email newsletter with tips to help you succeed in your health and fitness goals.

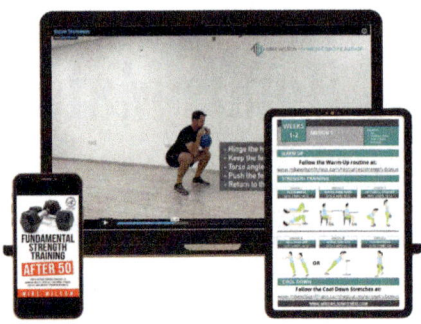

To get access to all this free bonus content; type in the link below into your chosen web browser or scan the QR code on the following page:

https://pages.mikewilsonfitness.com/strength-bonus

Scan the QR code below with your phone camera

Strength Training Bonus Material

Chapter 1

The "Simple Fitness After 50" Series

Let's take a reality check... our bodies naturally deteriorate as we age and this can have a profound effect on our lives if we let it.

Most people will notice subtle changes in their forties before it speeds up in their fifties and beyond. These changes can have multiple consequences on our lives; from struggling with simple tasks such as tying our shoelaces, right up to severe lack of functional capacity (our ability to do common daily tasks), pain and disease.

However, we have a choice. We can sit back and accept our destiny; our later years are going to be a regressive deterioration into a weak, immobile, painful version of ourselves. Or we can educate ourselves and take simple, actionable steps towards a better quality of life in our later years. By reading this book, I'm hoping the latter is your plan!

This is the first in a series of five books that will cover all the main components of fitness for the over 50s. The series aims to educate you on how you can implement changes in your life right now, to allow yourself to live your later years with more energy, perform activities of daily living with more ease, experience less pain and discomfort, have higher levels of self-confidence, self-esteem, and self-efficacy, and lower your risk of disease.

My decision to write a series of books covering *fitness after 50* is to allow you, as the reader, to focus on the fitness components that are more relevant to your needs rather than purchasing a general fitness book. Also, it comes down to my belief that to be in optimal health, both physically and mentally, beyond the age of fifty, it takes a multi-component approach rather than a single-component approach.

This belief is backed up by the 2018 PAGAC (Physical Activity Guidelines Advisory Committee) scientific report. The report provided strong evidence that a multi-component approach to fitness has greater improvements (compared to single-component) to physical function in older age, and is more likely to prevent falls and fall-related injuries.

I'm not implying that those in their 50s have a high risk of falls and fall-related injuries, but this is an obvious risk when in your 60s and beyond. Therefore, implementing appropriate fitness interventions in your 50s can not only allow you to become fit, strong, and healthy, and allow you to complete your last 10-15 years of your working life with more ease and ability, it also sets you up for a healthy lifestyle in your 60s and beyond.

Don't wait for the symptoms of aging to kick in and then attempt to *cure* them. Start training now and *prevent* those symptoms from kicking in for as long as possible!

The Simple Fitness After 50 Series:

Book 1: Fundamental Strength Training After 50

Book 2: Fundamental Core Training After 50 (Est. release date - July 2022)

Book 3: Fundamental Balance Training After 50 (Est. release date - October 2022)

Book 4: Fundamental Mobility and Flexibility After 50 (Est. release date - January 2023)

Book 5: Fundamental Posture Training After 50 (Est. release date - March 2023)

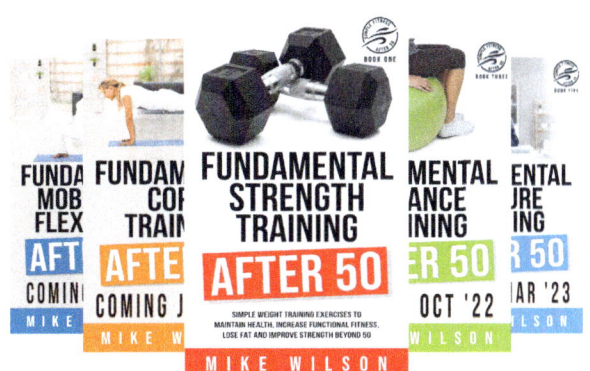

Simple Fitness After 50 Series

Chapter 2

Introduction

Strength training can be complex and confusing. There are hundreds of different exercises using various types of equipment. There is also a multitude of fitness 'gurus' claiming that they have the exact "method" to achieve YOUR results.

Regardless of what anyone says, there is no magic formula for achieving your results; it comes down to being consistent with effective methods that suit you, whilst applying some basic training principles.

The simpler and more manageable the training is, the more likely you will show long-term consistency and for strength training to become a habit. Not only that, but it's possible to achieve amazing results using just a few simple, fundamental movement patterns.

I have written this book to simplify becoming fit, strong and healthy, specifically for those beyond the age of fifty. For those whose time becomes more precious and goals become more orientated towards health, wellbeing, functional capabilities (work & home-life), life-longevity, and maintaining a body (and mind!) that is as youthful as possible, for as long as possible.

This is in contrast to the younger generation, who *may* have fewer health concerns, have not yet started any physical deterioration, and have more of an interest in appearance, impressing a potential partner, and/or sports.

The challenge of committing to a strength training program is hard enough as it is, but whether you plan to train at the gym or at home, the minefield of equipment and exercises can be mind-boggling, so what *should* you do?

You may have asked the advice of friends or family who are into health and fitness or appear in shape, and they all come up with different answers! The truth is, there is more than one way to achieve your goals, but the fundamentals of strength training after 50 stay the same:

(i) provide your body with a repetitive load that is greater than what your body is used to, (ii) perform multi-joint exercises utilizing large muscle groups, (iii) select exercises that are safe, effective, and promote good posture, and (iv) perform exercises that slow the aging process and aid your functional capacity.

You can improve your muscular health and fitness significantly by performing *'The Essential Eight'* fundamental movement patterns; *The Squat, The Hip Hinge, The Step Up, The Horizontal Pull, The Vertical Pull, The Horizontal Push, The Vertical Push,* and *The Carry.*

My plan is *not* to be one of those fitness professionals that provides you with an 'exact formula' for success. My plan is to simplify the entire process, with logical (and scientific) justification for my recommendations, to focus on the most fundamental human movement patterns and eliminate any exercises that are dysfunctional, less effective, time-consuming, high-risk, complicated and unnecessary.

I want to give you the most "bang for your buck" with your strength training; maximizing your results in the simplest, safest, and most time-efficient manner.

The Essential Eight will...

- Be simple enough to maximize consistency and adherence
- Use all major muscle groups in a balanced and functional program
- Minimize the risk of injuries associated with resistance training
- Enable you to increase muscular strength and/or endurance
- Maintain or improve your posture long term
- Increase basal metabolic rate (BMR); increasing daily energy expenditure & aiding long-term weight management
- Help you lose fat when combined with appropriate food consumption
- Be time-efficient, minimizing the impact on your lifestyle
- Increase your functional capacity and ability to perform activities of daily living (ADL)
- Help to maintain bone density throughout later-life
- Help reduce loss of muscle mass throughout later-life
- Reduce the risk of age-related health conditions

The Essential Eight is a simple but effective method of improving and maintaining your muscular fitness for the rest of your life.

Have fun and don't forget to use my exercise video library (see the webpage in the bonus material) to get more of a visual demonstration of how to perform the exercises safely and effectively.

Chapter 3

The Aging Process

The aging process involves natural degeneration of the body systems, including the three associated with human movement; the skeletal system, muscular system and nervous system. This degeneration can lead to a decrease in functional capacity from around the age of 50 onwards and can speed up in later life.

The following occur naturally to the human movement systems during the aging process:

- Muscle mass decreases. This is thought to occur at a rate of approximately 3-8% every 10 years from the age of 30, and at a higher rate from age 60. Age-related muscle loss is known as sarcopenia.
- Bone density decreases. This occurs at varying rates and begins at around the age of 50, but speeds up significantly in later life. This can lead to osteopenia and potentially osteoporosis.
- Balance deteriorates. Our ability to keep our centre of gravity over our base of support decreases with age, increasing the chance of falls and broken bones when associated with bone density loss.
- Coordination deteriorates. Our ability for the nervous system and muscular system to communicate efficiently decreases with age, making our movement patterns less controlled, which can

cause lower force output and potential loss of balance and increased falls.
- Connective tissue elasticity decreases. This can lead to reduced joint mobility, muscular flexibility, poor posture, and increased risk of injury.

The human movement systems affect every physical action we take; as they degenerate and weaken, it has a profound impact on basic functional capabilities such as carrying shopping bags, getting in and out of chairs, using stairs, and opening jars and tin cans.

Luckily for us, effective strength training can reduce the rate of deterioration, and help maintain our functional capacity in our later life.

Not only can strength training positively affect the degenerative processes outlined above, but it can also have an indirect impact on all body systems. For example, a lower metabolic rate accompanies a decrease in muscle mass and an increase in body fat. This can lead to obesity, type 2 diabetes, heart disease, joint problems, and more.

Strength training can maintain or even increase muscle mass in mid-later life. Therefore, it is likely to help maintain a healthy body composition (higher muscle mass and lower body fat) and reduce the risk of associated diseases.

Chapter 4

Strength Training Principles

It is common for people to perceive the term 'strength training' differently than other people, so let's clarify my meaning and terminology throughout this book.

Strength training includes the performance of any exercise that causes our muscles to contract and create a force to move a load or weight; either our body weight and/or a specific external load, such as a barbell, dumbbells, kettlebells, etc. Other terms given to this type of exercise are "resistance training" and "weight training". Generally, they mean the same thing.

Benefits of Strength Training After 50

It's never too late to experience the benefits of strength training. Those over 50 can benefit from strength training in multiple ways, including:

- Increased muscle mass
- Improved bone mass (density & content) and bone strength; decreasing the risk of osteoporosis
- Increased Resting Metabolic Rate; increasing energy expenditure and improved weight management
- Reduces excess body fat

- Increased functional capacity (your ability to carry out activities of daily living related to work and home life)
- Lower risk of developing functional limitations
- Lower risk of all-cause mortality
- Improved coordination, stability and balance
- Improved blood pressure in those who are pre-hypertensive or stage 1 hypertensive
- Increased self-confidence and self-efficacy
- Helps prevent falls

A multitude of studies have shown that regular strength training can significantly reduce the symptoms of age-related conditions, including:

- Arthritis
- Diabetes
- Lower back pain
- Osteoporosis
- Obesity
- Hyperlipidemia
- Dementia
- Depression

As well as these benefits of strength training, research shows that your functional capacity, which is your ability to perform activities of daily living (ADLs), improves with regular strength training.

A study conducted by Dr. Chiung-Ju Liu of Purdue University, Indianapolis, looked at 121 trials involving 6,700 participants in the age range 60-80. The research found that those who performed strength training activities 2-3 times per week consistently outperformed those that didn't on common daily movements such as getting out of a chair, and also showed a large positive effect on muscle strength.

Types of Strength Training

Methods of Strength Training are often classified by the type of load or resistance that is applied to the muscles.

Bodyweight

As the name suggests, this type of strength training uses the person's own weight as resistance. Push Ups, Dips, Chin Ups and Pull Ups are all forms of bodyweight exercises, and we can learn many more exercises by using our body weight before progressing to more challenging forms, such as Weighted Squats, Step Ups, and lunges.

Resistance Machines

Resistance Machines are commonly found in health clubs and gyms. They are very safe and enable a movement pattern to be learnt through a fixed path. However, they do not incorporate stabilizing muscles, including the core, and are bulky, expensive, and lack versatility. Examples include Leg Press Machine, Chest Press Machine, and Lat Pull Down Machine.

Cable Machines

Cable Machines are also commonly found in health clubs, gyms and also small fitness studios. They are again bulky and expensive, but much more versatile than resistance machines, allowing the path of movement and direction of resistance to be adjusted to suit various exercises. They also allow lots of movements/exercises to be performed from a standing position, making them particularly functional.

Free Weights

Free weights are types of equipment that can freely move in any direction. This means they require more stabilization from the user, have more versatility than resistance machines, are smaller and less expensive, but can have a steeper learning curve. They include barbells, dumbbells, and kettlebells.

Resistance Bands

Resistance bands are like large rubber bands, which provide resistance when stretched. They are inexpensive, light and portable, and versatile. You can purchase them in various resistance levels to suit different exercises and individuals. Resistance bands are not as freely moveable and have limited resistance compared to free weights.

Suspension Trainers

Suspension trainers, such as the TRX®, are essentially a pair of straps with one end that attaches to a fixed anchor point and handles at the other end. They are relatively inexpensive, light and portable, and versatile. They provide a high level of joint and core stabilization but are limited by the user's body weight and the need for a sturdy anchor point at an appropriate height.

Home-Based Strength Training Equipment

Many of you may wish to perform your strength training at home. If so, you will need to set yourself up with a small amount of equipment. This does not need to be of the commercial standards that you would find in a health club or gym, but I would suggest avoiding very cheap equipment as you may sacrifice on quality and increase the safety risk.

It may be a good idea to finish this book first before deciding on equipment, as you may decide that you can adapt to work with just a couple of pieces of equipment, rather than buying everything at once.

To help you out, I've created an equipment list for my recommendations below. Go to mikewilsonfitness.com/resources/equipment-list/ to access the equipment list.

Mat

These will provide support and cushioning when performing any floor-based exercises, as well as during any stretches that you perform after your training session.

Training Towel

You can place a towel between you and your mat/bench to protect your equipment from sweat, and also dry your hands between sets of exercises to prevent loss of grip. They are also useful for mopping your brow when you break a sweat!

Bench

A workout bench is a useful piece of equipment for lying and seated exercises, and can also provide support for other exercises such as the single-arm row. For more versatility and a lower price point, a "fitness deck" provides the benefits of a fitness step and bench all in one.

Dumbbells

As mentioned earlier, dumbbells are a form of free weight. They are versatile and an excellent option for improving joint stability, left/right muscle imbalances, coordination, and balance in older adults. Rather than buying an entire set of dumbbells like you would see in a health club or gym, you can purchase adjustable dumbbells that will be more affordable and space-saving.

Barbell & Plates

Barbells & plates are not essential, as you can perform all exercises with alternative equipment. They are also relatively bulky compared to other equipment. You may, however, choose to add them to your equipment list when you get stronger in exercises such as the deadlift and squat.

Kettlebells

Kettlebells are a brilliant piece of equipment for home-based training as they are relatively compact, versatile, and excellent for multi-joint movements. There is also one exercise that we'll look at later in the book, that can only be executed correctly using a kettlebell.

Resistance Bands

Resistance bands are very affordable, lightweight and portable, and very versatile. They are an excellent piece of equipment for home-based training but are unlikely to fulfil all your needs on a long-term basis.

Suspension Trainer

A suspension trainer, such as a TRX®, is great if you have some outside space with a suitable anchor point, or have a spacious indoor space where you can use a specialist door anchor. They are great for adding joint and core stabilization during strength training exercises, but will only be effective if you have the space and an anchor point, so research this before committing to purchasing one.

Are All Strength Training Exercises 'Good'?

I prefer to view exercises as more appropriate or less appropriate, rather than good or bad. This is because some exercises could be bad for some people and good for others. Therefore, it is not the case that an exercise was good or bad, one may be more appropriate for one person and a different exercise may be more appropriate for another person.

Based on the target readers of this book, people in their 50s, 60s, 70s, and maybe 80s, we will focus on one category of exercises known as compound exercises and will not be covering any exercises in the opposite category known as isolation exercises.

Compound Exercises

A compound exercise is one that involves multiple joints (usually 2 or 3) moving simultaneously. Upper body compound exercises usually involve the shoulder(s) and elbow(s) moving simultaneously, and lower body compound exercises usually involve the hip(s), knee(s), and ankle(s) moving simultaneously. Examples include Bench Press, Push Ups, Bent Over Row, Chin Ups, Squats and Step Ups, among others.

Isolation Exercises

An isolation exercise is one that involves a single moving joint (either on one side or both sides of the body). Upper body isolation exercises usually involve the shoulder(s) moving only, OR the elbow(s) moving only. Examples include Chest Fly, Reverse Fly, Side Raises, Bicep Curl, and Tricep Extension, among others. Lower body isolation exercises usually involve the hip(s) moving only, OR the knee(s) moving only, OR the ankle(s) moving only, Examples include: Standing Hip Extensions, Leg Extensions, Hamstring Curls, and Calf Raises, among others.

Compound Exercises vs. Isolation Exercises?

Most of the population would benefit from basing their strength training around compound exercises, but it is even more relevant to those over 50.

Compressional Forces vs Shear Forces

Compound exercises cause compressional forces where forces are applied from one end of long bones to the other. Long bones are located, among other places, in the arms and legs, which are the main moving body parts in daily life and exercise.

When a stimulus is applied to the body, the body adapts, especially if the stimulus is greater than what it's used to. Compressional forces are less likely to cause injury, and more likely to stimulate bone formation; decreasing the rate at which we lose bone density through the aging process.

Isolation exercises cause shear forces, where forces are applied *across* long bones. Shear forces are more likely to cause injury and stimulate bone formation to a lesser extent than compressional forces.

Winner = Compound Exercises

Lever Length and Risk of Injury

The limbs (arms and legs) act as levers during many exercises. Lever length is the distance between the moving joint and the weight in the hands. The lever length, as well as the load (e.g. dumbbell), determine how much force is applied to the moving joint. The longer the lever is, the greater the stress is placed on the moving joint, causing a higher risk of injury.

Compound exercises utilize short lever lengths, isolation exercises utilize greater lever lengths. Therefore, compound = lower risk of injury, isolation = higher risk of injury.

Winner = Compound Exercises

Time Efficiency

Compound exercises involve multiple joints, and therefore more muscle groups and greater overall muscle mass than isolation exercises that involve one moving joint. This means that compound exercises make your workouts more time-efficient; you could achieve a full-body workout in as little as three exercises, whereas it could take eight or more isolation exercises to achieve a full-body workout.

Winner = Compound Exercises

Muscle Mass, Force Output and Hormonal Response

With multiple joints moving, and more muscle groups involved, compound exercises allow you to produce more force output and therefore lift a heavier load when compared to isolation.

This causes a greater hormonal response from your endocrine system, particularly elevated levels of testosterone and growth hormones post-training. This aids tissue (muscle) formation and growth, slowing or reversing age-related losses of muscle mass.

Winner = Compound Exercises

Functionality

The word "functional" gets used a lot in the fitness industry, probably too much! The level of functionality of an exercise depends on how closely it replicates movements that are performed in daily life or sport.

There is often a lot of debate about whether an exercise is "functional", or whether one exercise is more functional than another. We will not be debating the minor details of this across specific exercises, but compound exercises are always more functional than isolation exercises.

When we move in daily life and sport, we are required to produce a force output for desired tasks. Our aim is to produce the force in the most efficient manner possible, which is best done by recruiting a large amount of muscle mass spread across multiple joints.

Many tasks would be impossible, or at least look silly if we aimed to perform them by moving one joint only. For example, imagine climbing your stairs without the ability to move your hips, knees and ankle simultaneously! Or getting up from a chair without moving your knees!

Winner = Compound Exercises

Coordination

Coordination degenerates with age. The more we keep our neuromuscular system (nervous system and muscular system) active and challenged, the slower the degeneration will be.

Compound exercises require the nervous system to communicate with many muscles simultaneously to produce multiple joint movements with the desired magnitude (force and direction), resulting in a coordinated movement pattern.

During isolation exercises, the demand placed on the neuromuscular system is less because of the single joint and lesser muscle recruitment required. The greater the demand placed upon the neuromuscular system, the more coordination will be maintained or improved.

Winner = Compound Exercises

Summary

Isolation exercises are not bad exercises, but they are less appropriate for those over 50.

They can be great for increasing muscle mass in specific muscles, can create variety and interest for those wanting to spend hours in the gym, can aid rehabilitation from injury, and can be programmed for specific postural correction.

If you don't have a specific reason for including isolation exercises, it's best to stick to compound exercises.

Compound exercises are the most appropriate category of strength training exercises to slow the aging process and live a healthier later life, with greater functional capacity and lower risk of injury and disease.

Training Terminology

Repetitions (Reps): how many times you perform an exercise. '10 reps' means that the exercise is performed 10 times before stopping and resting.

Sets: a set is a group of repetitions. 2 sets of 10 reps = 10 reps - rest - 10 reps - exercise finished.

Load: the 'weight' of the equipment that the muscles are producing force against. E.g. weight of barbells or dumbbells.

Rest: the time taken to rest and recover between sets.

Hypertrophy Training: resistance training performed using specific variables (sets/repetitions/load/rest) to maximize the increase in the size of muscles.

Endurance Training: resistance training performed using specific variables (sets/repetitions/load/rest) to maximize the ability of muscles to perform repeated efforts with minimal fatigue.

Chapter 5

Habit vs Quick Fix

The key to gaining and maintaining lifelong health and fitness is making physical activity a habit; part of your lifestyle rather than a short-term quick-fix.

By focusing on the key fundamentals and keeping exercise simple, it becomes time-efficient, makes it easier to focus on the goal in-hand, creates increased consistency, and has a higher chance of being seamlessly incorporated into your current lifestyle.

To enable you to get from a relatively sedentary lifestyle to a point where exercise is a regular and consistent habit, I recommend focusing some time on effective goal setting.

When asked about goals, most clients would respond with comments such as "I want to lose weight" or "I want to get stronger/fitter".

The problem with these 'goals' is that they are too vague and probably not the deep-rooted goal. They are too vague because if a person spends a year exercising to lose weight, and after 12 months they have lost 1lb, they have essentially achieved the goal of losing weight! However, 1lb over 12 months probably wasn't what they hoped for. Therefore, goals need to be much more specific and detailed.

In terms of not being the 'deep-rooted' goal, when a person says they want to lose weight it usually isn't the weight loss they want, it's what accompanies the weight loss... the emotions and feelings it creates such as increased self-confidence and happiness in one's self.

People rarely want to get stronger or fitter for the sake of it, it's the ability to do activities or tasks with more ease, to a higher level, without getting breathless or aching. Simple things like using the stairs, playing with the children/grandchildren, walking to enjoy some sightseeing, or playing a sport to a higher level.

Simply saying you want to lose weight or get stronger is like saying you want to earn more money without having a "why" (have a nicer house, new car, travel more, etc.). It's the "why" that becomes the motivational driver for achieving the goal, not the actual goal itself.

To help you set goals effectively, I want you to do *four things*:

1. Set a combination of outcome goals and process goals.
2. Use the SMART acronym for setting Specific, Measurable, Achievable, Relevant, and Time-Bound goals.
3. Set short, medium, and long-term goals.
4. Write a list of WHY you want to achieve your goals. Write them or use an image to represent them, and have them on your computer background, on a notice board in your house, on the fridge, or wherever is highly visible on a daily basis. Focus on these regularly, particularly when you hit a point in the journey where you are struggling to adhere to your training.

Outcome vs Process Goals

An outcome goal is an *end result*, whereas process goals are things that will be put in place to achieve the outcome. For example, if the outcome goal is to lose 3cm from the waist by the end of month 3, then a process goal could be to reduce daily calorie consumption by 10% for the next 3 months. The waist circumference reduction is the *outcome/result*. One *process* to achieve this is to reduce daily calorie consumption by 10%.

SMART Goals

- Specific
- Measurable
- Achievable
- Relevant
- Time-Bound

Specific

This is where you need to add details. "I want to lose weight" vs "I will lose 10lb and reduce my waist circumference by 2cm". Note not only the detail added but the change in the verb from 'want' to 'will'. The former suggests it's a desire, a hope, that you will achieve it. The latter is a statement of intent, confirmation that it is going to happen. "I will…" is a more powerful statement than "I want…".

Measurable

You need to be able to track progress and have a clear indication of whether a goal was achieved or not.

It needs to be quantifiable, with no room for misinterpretation or guesswork. By adding the amount of weight loss (e.g. 10lb), assuming you take a baseline measurement before starting, you can weigh yourself periodically (I don't suggest more regularly than every 1-2 weeks) to track progress and know if you lost the 10lb or not.

If you are unsure how you will measure progress and the result, you either need to change the goal, add more detail, or find a method of measuring it using an appropriate fitness test (See *Chapter 7: Tracking Progress* for some examples).

Achievable

Think carefully about the amount/quantities associated with your goal and ensure that they are challenging but achievable. If it's not a challenge, your focus and determination are likely to fade. If your goal is so extreme that it's unachievable, then you are setting yourself up for failure from day 1. It needs to require some hard work, but be realistic.

Relevant

Many people use the 'R' in SMART as 'realistic' but this usually comes under the term achievable, so I want you to ensure that every goal is relevant to the overall outcome you are trying to achieve.

For example, if your overall outcome goal is to improve your strength to perform daily tasks with more ease, then a goal to run 5km 3x/week isn't relevant unless you have some kind of aerobic fitness goal as well. "I will complete a 30-minute total-body strength training session, 3 times per week" is a relevant *process goal* to the overall *outcome goal*.

Time-Bound

All goals are a distant ambition unless you give yourself a deadline for outcome goals and a time and frequency for process goals.

If we take the earlier goal of "I will lose 10lb and reduce my waist circumference by 2cm", we simply need to add a deadline to make it time-bound.

"I will lose 10lb and reduce my waist circumference by 2cm, by the end of (month/year)" is now a SMART goal; it has details, it is quantifiable and measurable via weighing scales and a tape measure, it is achievable if based on a short-medium timeframe such as 2 months, it would be relevant to the person, and it is time-bound.

Short, Medium and Long-term Goals

Setting goals with various timeframes help to keep you focused and achieve smaller results on the journey to a bigger result. It helps create a positive experience (when goals are SMART) and aids in exercise adherence (sticking to the exercise plan!).

I would suggest that short-term goals can be anything between 1 week and 1 month, medium-term goals are anything between 1 and 3 months, and long-term goals are anything between 3 and 12 months.

Chapter 6

Health Screening

Health Screening is the process of determining whether you are in a healthy enough condition to start a new exercise program.

All exercise puts additional short-term stresses on the body, and it's your responsibility to determine whether you are healthy enough to cope with those additional stresses.

I will outline what is required to perform the health screening process below, but if in any doubt, seek advice from a medical professional before commencing any new exercise program.

Physical Activity Readiness Questionnaire (PAR-Q)

The standard tool used to determine whether an individual is healthy enough to start an exercise program is the Physical Activity Readiness Questionnaire (PAR-Q). I highly recommend that you complete the PAR-Q for Everyone form at the PAR-Q+ website (eparmedx.com) before commencing any new physical activity program.

Physical Activity Readiness Questionnaire

Resting Blood Pressure

I recommend taking this test prior to starting an exercise program. It is a key indicator of the health of your heart. To take your blood pressure, you will need a basic blood pressure monitor, and follow the included instructions.

You always get two readings:

Systolic BP = pressure on the artery walls when the heart pushes blood into the arteries

Diastolic BP: pressure on the artery walls between heart contractions

It's always given as systolic BP "over" diastolic BP.

120/80 = 120 "over" 80 = a systolic BP of 120 (mmHg) and diastolic BP of 80 (mmHg).

A healthy blood pressure reading should be between 90/60 and 120/80. If you fit into this category, then it would suggest your cardiovascular system is healthy enough to start an exercise program, assuming your PAR-Q and resting heart rate are also giving this outcome.

If your blood pressure is above 120/80 but below 140/90, then it is slightly higher than you'd want it to be and is known as "pre-hypertensive". In this case, it's a good idea to implement some lifestyle changes to reduce it, and monitor it over the following few months until it lowers into the 90/60 - 120/80 range.

If your blood pressure is above 140/90 (at rest) then you are hypertensive (you have high BP). Only your GP/Physician can provide confirmation and 'diagnosis' of this, so don't presume you are hypertensive based on your readings. You may not truly be at rest, therefore it could just be a temporary reading, and/or there may be some error in your equipment or the use of it.

Based on your age (over 50) and your BP being over 140/90, I recommend seeking advice from your GP/Physician before commencing your program. If it's above 140/90 but below 160/100 there should be no reason for them to advise against exercise, but it may involve pursuing with caution with specific guidance including:

- Extend your warm ups and cool downs, and perform them more gradually.
- Include some steady-state aerobic exercise in your weekly routine.
- Ensure you breathe correctly during strength training exercises (see Chapter 10)
- Avoid lifting weight above your head.
- Avoid jumping/bounding activities.
- Progress weights/load gradually.
- Avoid pushing to maximal effort.
- Work one side of the body (left/right) at a time (only really necessary if over 160/100).

If your blood pressure is above 160/100, the GP/Physician may recommend that you delay starting a strength training program until it has lowered, either through medication or, preferably, through nutritional changes and introducing some aerobic exercise.

If your blood pressure is below 90/60, then you are hypotensive (you have low blood pressure). If this applies to you, I would suggest seeking advice from your GP/Physician prior to starting the exercise program. Assuming there is no medical condition causing it, there should be no reason you cannot exercise, but you may need to transition between lying and standing with caution, as it may cause temporary dizziness.

Resting Heart Rate

I also recommend taking this test prior to starting an exercise program. It is another key indicator of the health of your heart, and although this book is about strength training rather than aerobic/cardio training, I recommend checking this prior to starting any new exercise/training program.

To measure your resting heart rate, either find your radial pulse (wrist) or carotid pulse (neck) and count how many beats you can feel over 60 seconds. Ensure you have been sitting down (or laying) and feeling relaxed for 5+ minutes before taking it, preferably when you wake in the morning.

A normal resting heart rate is between 60 and 100 beats per minute (bpm). Resting heart rate increases because of the aging process, but should remain within this range.

If you have a resting heart rate of 100 bpm or more, it is known as tachycardia, and you must see your GP/Physician before commencing an exercise program.

If your resting heart rate is below 100 bpm, and assuming no other tests, including the PAR-Q, imply otherwise, it would suggest your heart is sufficiently healthy to start an exercise program.

A healthier heart has a lower resting heart rate (within reason). A low resting heart rate suggests a strong heart capable of pumping a high volume of blood into the arteries, requiring fewer beats/contractions per minute.

A resting heart rate below 60 bpm is known as bradycardia. It is possible that people have a resting heart rate, especially when asleep, of between 40 and 60 bpm and has no adverse effect on health. This is especially common in younger, healthy adults and trained athletes.

If you have a resting heart rate under 60 and experience dizziness, weakness, unusual tiredness or shortness of breath, ensure you see a GP/Physician before starting an exercise program.

Chapter 7

Tracking Progress

Importance of Tracking Progress

As much as we would all love the results from our training and exercise to happen overnight, they don't! They occur gradually over several weeks and months, potentially years, depending on the size of your goal(s)!

If you could take a sneak preview of how you would look and feel in 6 months' time, you would hopefully see and feel a big difference (for the better). But this big change would be the accumulation of small daily and weekly changes.

When the changes are small, you don't notice them yourself, and those closest to you may not notice them either. This is because your mind and body are adapting constantly to the slight changes and each week you become the 'newest version of yourself'; your new normal.

It's the people that don't see you for 6 months that will be shocked and comment on how you've changed.

If you don't notice your body changing, you may believe that your training and exercise aren't having a positive impact and give up, when actually you were making slight changes that would have accumulated into a big long-term change.

Tracking progress allows you to monitor your changes over time, giving you objective data as regular feedback on your progress. This helps you to adhere to the training long term, boost motivation, and also see if any changes you've made have helped or hindered progress.

How to Track Progress

You can track progress in several ways. It's imperative that you choose methods that apply to your goals. If you want to lose body fat, there's no point in monitoring your bench press 1 rep max!

Once you've chosen relevant methods to track progress, you must create some baseline measurements. This means doing the chosen tests prior to starting your journey. The results from these tests don't have any value at that moment in time, but they are your reference points for the future.

Many people get caught up in whether the results from the tests are 'good' or 'bad' and hope they compare to others. That's not what's important. You're aiming to be the best version of yourself, so take those initial measurements as baseline figures and then, in the future, you can compare the newest version of yourself to the older version of yourself.

Validity and Reliability

You need to ensure that any test is valid.

This means that it measures what it's actually supposed to measure. For example, if you are aiming to reduce body fat percentage and you simply weighed yourself regularly, the progress tracking is not valid because the weighing scales cannot distinguish between fat, muscle, bone, organs and other soft tissue. So the test is monitoring overall body weight, not body fat alone.

The tests also need to be reliable.

This means that you need to be able to repeat the test over time with no variables changing the outcome.

For example, weighing yourself on different scales is not reliable. The change in equipment, which has a certain margin of error, has introduced a variable that may change the outcome regardless of whether you lost or gained weight.

Another example; you measure your baseline resting blood pressure first thing in the morning, prior to breakfast, showering, and getting dressed. The next time you take the measurement, you have just got home from a long day at work, during which you consumed several cups of coffee, and got stuck in traffic on the way home. This is not reliable. There are several variables that will change the result regardless of any improvements in heart health.

Health & Fitness Tests

Before choosing the tests to perform, ensure you have performed your goal setting effectively, thinking deeply about what it really is you want to achieve.

Body Weight

Weighing yourself on weighing scales provides you with your total body weight. If you have significant weight to lose, then it can be a valid and reliable test for overall weight loss.

If your goals are more oriented towards fat loss and a change in body composition (fat mass vs lean body mass), then weighing is not a valid indicator of progress, and therefore is best avoided.

If you choose to use body weight to monitor progress, I advise you to weigh every 1-2 weeks. Never more frequently than that.

The reason for this is that weight loss *never* decreases linearly over time. If you lost 9kg over a 90-day period, that would be an average of 0.1kg (100g) per day. If you weighed every day for that 90-day period, I can guarantee that you will not be 0.1kg lighter each day.

You would find that some days it may appear that you lost some weight, other days it may appear that nothing changed, and other days it would appear that you put on weight! This inconsistency in progress, and seeing days where you supposedly put on weight or didn't lose any, are disheartening, frustrating, and demoralizing.

This could easily lead to you believing that your new lifestyle isn't helping you to achieve your goals and you give up and return to your old ways. Little did you know that if you stuck with it, it would've (theoretically) resulted in a 9kg loss of weight over the 90 days!

Use weighing scales with caution! If you cannot stop yourself from jumping on them, throw them out!!

Body Mass Index (BMI)

BMI is often used by government and health service studies to show whether a population is considered to be underweight, normal weight, overweight, or obese.

It is a value that is derived from both your weight and your height. It is calculated by dividing your weight in kilograms by your height in metres squared (kg/m^2).

The following table illustrates the categories of BMI:

BMI Classification	
Underweight	<18.5
Normal range	18.5-24.9
Overweight	25-29.9
Obese (Class I)	30-34.9
Obese (Class II)	35-39.9
Obese (Class III)	≥40.0

Body Mass Index Classifications

As it's a commonly used indicator of health by health professionals, it's worth calculating your BMI. However, when used alone, it can be an inaccurate measure of health because it does not take your body composition into consideration.

For example, two people can both weigh 95kg and have a height of 1.8m, giving them the same BMI of 29.3 (overweight, close to obese). Despite this, one of these could have relatively large muscle mass, low levels of body fat, low waist circumference, and consequently a low risk of disease. The other could have relatively little muscle mass, high levels of body fat, a large waist circumference, and consequently, a high risk of disease. In this instance, the BMI is likely a good indicator of health for the latter individual, but not the former.

Circumference Measurements

Circumference measurements involve measuring and monitoring the circumference of body parts such as the upper arms, chest, waist, hips, thighs, and lower leg. This is a better method of monitoring fat loss than weighing scales and is also great for monitoring hypertrophy (increases in muscle size).

It is a misconception that muscle weighs more than fat. If you have 1kg of fat and 1kg of muscle, they both weigh the same! The important factor is the density and therefore the space they take up in your body.

Fat has a relatively low density and therefore is relatively large; taking up a lot of space in the body and making you appear large and/or overweight. Muscle has a relatively high density and is therefore relatively small; taking up a smaller amount of space in the body and making you appear slim/lean/athletic.

Two people can weigh exactly the same, but one of those people can appear much larger and "overweight" than the other. This person's mass is taken up by a large proportion of fat, whereas the person's mass who doesn't appear to be overweight is taken up by a larger proportion of muscle (and less fat). This affects circumference measurements.

If a person who has a relatively large amount of body fat, appearing overweight, takes part in strength training (and other relevant training) their circumference measurements are likely to decrease as the less dense, *space-hogging* body fat reduces due to increased energy expenditure (exercise and resting metabolic rate due to increased muscle mass and active muscle mass).

As muscle is denser and relatively smaller, the reduction in fat will be greater than the gain in muscle mass and circumference measurements will decrease. This is great for tracking and monitoring progress.

If you have low levels of body fat and wish to focus on increased muscle mass and strength, circumference measurements are still a great way to monitor your progress. As muscle size increases and body fat doesn't change significantly, the resulting measurements should increase.

This could be more complex. It may not be about overall weight loss/fat loss/muscle gain. It may be more about body shape. Here are a couple of examples:

- You may wish to decrease the circumference of your waist (by reducing body fat) but increase the circumference of your chest and arms (by increasing muscle mass), or...
- You may wish to decrease the circumference of your waist and thighs (by reducing body fat), but increase the circumference of the hips (bum/glutes) (by increasing muscle mass).

Either way, circumference measurements work to track the progress of changes in body size and body shape, even when aiming for opposite results at different body parts.

If your goals are more oriented towards keeping up with the children/grandchildren, performing daily tasks with more ease, or feeling more confident in yourself; consider using circumference measurements if you believe that a change in muscle mass, fat mass, and/or body shape would aid these goals. If not, there is no need to measure or track them.

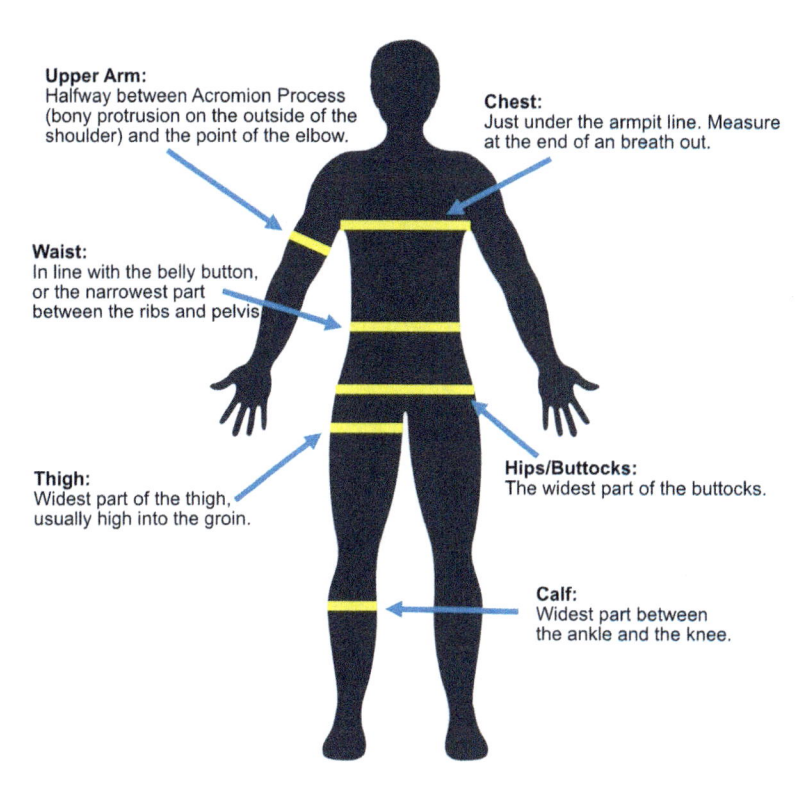

Upper Arm: Halfway between Acromion Process (bony protrusion on the outside of the shoulder) and the point of the elbow.

Chest: Just under the armpit line. Measure at the end of an breath out.

Waist: In line with the belly button, or the narrowest part between the ribs and pelvis.

Thigh: Widest part of the thigh, usually high into the groin.

Hips/Buttocks: The widest part of the buttocks.

Calf: Widest part between the ankle and the knee.

Circumference Measurement Sites

Waist Circumference

Waist circumference is often used as a key risk indicator of coronary heart disease and diabetes and is therefore worth monitoring, regardless of whether you use other circumference measurements outlined above.

Waist Circumference Classification				
Males		Females	
<94cm(37")	Low risk	<80cm(31.5")	Low risk
94cm(37") - 102cm(40")	High risk	80cm(31.5") - 88cm(34.6")	High risk
>102cm(40")	Very high risk	>88cm(34.6")	Very high risk

Waist Circumference Classification

To measure your waist circumference:

1. Find the bottom of your ribs and the top of your hips.
2. Place a tape measure around your middle at a point halfway between them (usually in line with or just above the belly button).
3. Make sure the tape measure is pulled tight, but isn't digging into your skin.
4. Breathe out naturally and take your measurement.
5. Take your measurement a second time, just to be sure.

Body Composition

Body composition is the percentage of your body that comprises lean body mass (muscle, bone, etc.) vs fat mass (visceral and subcutaneous body fat).

It is difficult and expensive to get a very accurate reading. Methods of measuring body composition usually come under one of two categories: 1) Accurate but expensive and/or inaccessible, or 2) Affordable, accessible, but inaccurate.

DEXA and MRI are medical scans that can provide accurate body composition but are expensive and inaccessible to most.

The most commonly used in fitness environments are a type of weighing scale with two separate metal plates. This is called bioelectrical impedance; it uses a weak electrical current to send through your body from one metal plate through the body to the other metal plate.

Muscle holds a high volume of the body's water content. Muscle and water give low resistance to the electrical impulse, whereas body fat provides high resistance. This enables the device to estimate body composition based on the amount of impedance (resistance) to the electrical impulse, affecting the voltage output.

There are a few major flaws to bioelectrical impedance:

- Electrical impulses take the shortest route from one metal plate to the other. If only your feet are on metal plates, the electrical impulse is only measuring impedance (resistance) in each leg. This doesn't factor in the body fat distribution as it's not measured around key areas such as the belly.
- Hydration levels impact results. This is not just affected by your water intake, but also your food consumption (amount/timing/food types), activity levels prior to measurement, caffeine consumption, etc.

One other commonly used method is the use of skin-fold calipers to measure the 'pinch' of skin and fat at specific anatomical landmarks. This method, if performed using high-quality calipers and an experienced professional, can be relatively accurate. But can also be fairly inaccurate if using cheap calipers by an inexperienced user.

My advice: don't worry about exact body composition. Circumference measurements are easier to perform accurately, using a very affordable device. Although it doesn't provide exact body composition measurements, it provides changes in body size, which indicates changes in muscle mass vs body fat.

Muscular Strength

The principal topic of this book is strength training, but that doesn't mean your goal is to increase your muscular strength. Of course, strength training is likely to make you stronger, but that is just one of many training outcomes of strength training. In fact, the adaptations that the muscular system makes in response to strength training can vary depending upon the number of repetitions (reps) performed in a set, and the corresponding load that is lifted.

There are 3 main primary outcomes on the muscular system:

Muscular Strength: This is the ability of the muscular system to overcome very large loads, just once or a few times. High levels of muscular strength result in the ability to move very heavy loads. However, it is not a measure of how many times you can move the load.

Someone who has high levels of muscular strength can lift very heavy objects, even if it's just once. But they are not usually very good at lifting lighter weights many times as they fatigue quickly.

To improve muscular strength, you need to lift very heavy weights with low repetitions, typically 1-5 reps.

Hypertrophy: This outcome is regarding the increase in the size of muscles. This outcome applies to most people as it increases resting metabolic rate, which increases daily energy expenditure (burns more calories daily), resulting in increased fat loss. It also optimizes body shape, is safer than training for muscular strength, and will still result in increased strength and all the benefits that come with that.

To improve muscular hypertrophy, you need to lift moderate to heavy weights (relative to you) with moderate repetitions, typically 6-12 reps. Progress is usually monitored via circumference measurements, outlined above.

Muscular Endurance: This is the ability of the muscular system to overcome relatively light loads repeatedly. Someone who has high levels of muscular endurance has a high resistance to fatigue when performing a movement against load many times. But they are not usually very good at lifting very heavy weights even for a few repetitions.

To improve muscular endurance, you need to lift light-moderate weights with high repetitions, typically >12.

Based on the above information, if you feel you need to track your progress in muscular strength, you simply need to measure and monitor the maximal load/weight you can perform on a select number of exercises.

Many athletes would perform a 1 rep max; record the maximum weight they can lift just once. This has a high risk of injury for a non-athlete, even one who has youth on their side, so I do not recommend it for the over 50s. I would suggest a 5 rep max on a Bench Press and Back Squat, and only for relatively well-conditioned older adults.

It is likely that testing and monitoring muscular strength is unnecessary for most readers of this book, so skip it unless you feel it's necessary for you, and you believe you are currently sufficiently conditioned to perform it.

Muscular Endurance

We've outlined above what muscular endurance is, and again, it is unlikely that you feel it is worthy of testing and monitoring. However, if you think it applies to your goals and you would benefit from testing it and monitoring it, here are two tests you can try:

Maximal Squat Test:

Find a chair or bench low enough to cause your knees to bend to 90° when you sit on the edge. Stand in front of it with your back to it. Squat down until your buttocks lightly touch the chair/bench and stand back up to a fully upright position. Repeat until you can no longer perform anymore and record the number of repetitions completed.

Aim for approximately 2s to complete each repetition to keep conditions consistent. Check bodyweight squat technique later on in the book before attempting this.

Maximal Push Up Test:

Choose either a full push up or ¾ push up. Check technique later in the book. Perform as many repetitions until you can no longer continue without rest. For repetitions to count, you must lower yourself until your elbows are at 90° and push all the way up, leaving only a slight bend in your elbow at the top. Aim for 2s per repetition. This will keep conditions consistent each time you attempt it. Record the number of reps performed.

Progress Photos

This is a test I highly recommend, along with circumference measurements. The circumference measurements give you the data in numbers/figures, and the photos give you the visual reference. Without them, you have no visual reference to compare your results against the earlier version of yourself.

After 6 months of training, you'll have got used to the new you, and won't know how significant your physical changes have been unless you can do a visual comparison.

Choose a location with good natural light and a plain background. Wear as minimal clothing as you're comfortable with (you choose who sees them!), stand in a relaxed state and take three photos; one facing the camera, one side on, and one with your back to the camera.

The first set of photos has no real immediate value. Save them somewhere safe, ready for when you do the next set of photos. Leave a minimum of 6 weeks between photos, and no more than 12 weeks.

Chapter 8

Myths & Misconceptions

Society may suggest that strength training is for the young. Strength Training is for everyone, as long as the level/difficulty is pitched appropriately to the individual.

The reason for performing strength training often changes with age, with the young focused more on aesthetics and/or sports performance, and older adults more focused on health and activities of daily living (ADL's), as well as potentially some aesthetics and sports performance.

There has been extensive research into strength training for older adults, and the positives of strength training far outweigh the negatives for those without significant and relevant health conditions.

Common Myths

"Strength Training isn't safe for older adults."

There's a misconception that beyond a certain age, you will be limited by your deteriorating physical capabilities, and this just needs to be accepted. The aging process happens. Nothing can change that. But strength training can delay it, slow it, enable you to manage it, and ultimately allow you to live a life with more energy, less fatigue, more capabilities, less pain, and improve your overall quality of life.

Strength training is safe as long as basic guidelines are adhered to; perform exercises with good technique, progress gradually, and work within your own limitations.

"Strength training is not a suitable form of exercise for older adults."

Based on the information provided in the chapter on the aging process and the benefits of strength training, I hope you can see how important strength training is to the health, well-being, and quality of life of older adults. I am not suggesting strength training is the ONLY form of exercise that is necessary, but it is one component of fitness that should not be ignored.

"Exercising and trying to be more healthy is pointless after 50, the decline in old age is inevitable"

This is simply not true. There are people in their 50s, 60s, 70s, and even 80's who are fitter than they have ever been. Some running marathons and becoming bodybuilders! Alicia I. Arbaje, MD, MPH, an assistant professor of Geriatrics and Gerontology at Johns Hopkins University School of Medicine in Baltimore, states that a lot of the symptoms that we associate with old age, such as weakness and loss of balance, are actually symptoms of inactivity, not age.

"It's too late to start exercising and make a difference to my health."

Studies have found that even people who start an exercise routine in their 90s can boost muscle strength. Further research shows that starting exercise late in life can still reduce the risk of health problems such as diabetes, and improve symptoms of such diseases. Dr. Chhanda Dutta, Chief of the Clinical Gerontology Branch, Division of Geriatrics and Clinical Gerontology, National Institute on Aging states that "it really is never too late to start exercising and reaping the benefits".

"Older adults should not perform strength training without the supervision of a health professional."

I'm a big advocate for supervised fitness training. Working in fitness education, including training people to become fitness instructors and personal trainers, has been a huge part of my 20+ years working in the fitness industry. I highly recommend you seek the advice and support of a well-respected personal trainer to further enhance your chances of achieving your desired results in a safe and timely manner. But personal training is not a necessity to achieve results.

I recommend seeing your GP/Physician prior to starting a strength training program and listening to their guidance and advice based on your age and health. But, assuming the GP/Physician has not advised against strength training, then unsupervised participation is perfectly reasonable, just like a younger person. As always, maintain excellent technique, work within your limitations, and progress gradually.

"Exercise cannot be good for me, it causes joint pain"

Chronic pain caused by arthritis, may mean exercising seems too painful. However, studies carried out on older adults with arthritis, show that regular exercise helps to reduce pain and improve joint function.

Chapter 9

Warm Up and Cool Down

Warm Up & Dynamic Stretches

Before performing any of your strength training exercises, it's important to perform an effective warm up to:

- Increase blood flow to the muscles
- Move muscles through their full range of motion
- Mobilize joints
- Stretch tight muscles
- Practice movement patterns without weight

The warm up should:

- Last 5-10 minutes
- Be progressive (gradually increase in intensity)
- Include multi-joint activities that increase the heart rate
- Involve dynamic stretches to mobilize joints and stretch muscles

Example Warm Up:

1. Walking (increasing speed or incline) - 2 mins
2. Marching (on spot) - 30s
3. High Knees - 30s
4. Jogging (on the spot if needed) - 1-2 mins
5. Arm Circles - 20s each arm
6. Chest Openers - 20s
7. Overhead Reach - 20s
8. Hip Circles - 20s each direction
9. Bodyweight squats - 30s
10. Side Lunges - 30s

You can gain access to a video demonstration of a comprehensive Warm Up by using the bonus material link at the beginning of this book.

Cool Down & Static Stretches

After you have completed your strength training, it's important to aid your recovery by performing a cool down and static stretch to:

- Gradually return the heart back towards a resting state to avoid any sudden changes
- Increase venous return (the blood flow from working muscles back to the heart)
- Avoid feeling dizzy
- Increase removal of waste products that may have built up in the muscles
- Lengthen muscles to avoid strength training, causing a loss in flexibility
- Release tension from working muscles
- Reduce post-training muscle soreness (DOMS - Delayed Onset Muscle Soreness)

The cool down and stretch should:

- Last 5-10 minutes
- Be regressive (gradually decrease in intensity)
- Involve multi-joint activities, with emphasis on movement in the legs
- Involve static stretches to return muscles to their resting length

Example Cool Down and Stretch:

1. Jogging, fast walking or cycling (decreasing speed/incline/intensity) - 3 mins
2. Stretch each major muscle group for 15s
    - Back
    - Chest
    - Glutes (bum)
    - Hamstrings (back of thigh)
    - Quadriceps (front of thigh)
    - Calves (back of lower leg)

You can gain access to a video demonstration of a full body static stretch routine by using the bonus material link at the beginning of this book.

Chapter 10

General Exercise Technique

Regardless of the exercise, there are some techniques that remain throughout all exercises. Let's have a look at them now before we get into the specifics of each exercise.

Spinal Alignment

The spine has 4 main curves, 3 of which can change significantly as we move. The aim is to keep a "neutral spine" (natural curves) through all strength training, to maximize the safety and effectiveness of the exercises.

A neutral spine has a slight inward/concave curve in the lower back (the lumbar vertebrae), and slight outward/convex curve in the upper back (the thoracic vertebrae), and another inward/concave curve in the back of the neck (the cervical vertebrae).

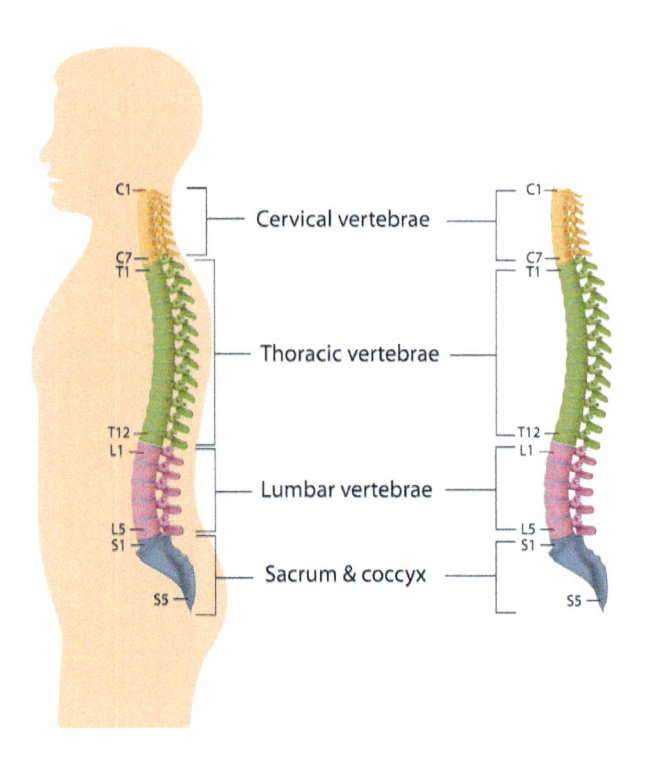

Curves & Sections of the Spine

To maintain a neutral spine, you can incorporate a few techniques before it becomes second nature:

1. Set the Pelvis. Tilt your pelvis all the way back, then all the way forward and then find an approximate mid-point. Imagine your pelvis as a bucket of water... tip the water out of the back, tip the water out of the front, then find a midpoint so no water tips out!
2. Engage your core. Create a slight hollowing of your belly by drawing inwards towards your lower spine. Make this subtle, so you can still breathe normally. Engage your pelvic floor by imagining you are slowing or stopping the flow when you go for a pee!

3. Keep your chest proud. Lift your chest slightly and set your shoulder blades back and down into your back pockets (imaginary ones if need be!).
4. Bring your ears back in line with your shoulders and look straight ahead (when standing upright). Think about the gap between your chin and chest... keep that same gap regardless of what position/angle your torso is at during exercises.

Hip-Knee-Ankle (H-K-A) Alignment

Particularly relevant to lower body strength training exercises, aim to keep your knee joint inline between your hip and ankle. The easiest way to do this is to focus on the knee tracking in line with your 2nd and 3rd toes.

Wrist Alignment

Particularly relevant to upper body strength training exercises, aim to keep your wrist in a neutral position to avoid excess stresses on the joint. This is best achieved by ensuring you wrap your thumb around the bar you're holding, and point your knuckles (the ones halfway along your fingers) in the direction of the movement.

Range of Motion (ROM)

Range of motion, or range of movement, is the distance moved between the start and finish positions of each exercise. This is specific to each exercise, but there are a couple of cues to aid the achievement.

Keep joints, particularly elbows and knees, unlocked at the end range of motion, rather than locking them out. At the other end of the range of motion, ensure all body parts and joints stay in alignment, specific to that exercise.

Tempo

Tempo is the speed at which you move during the exercise.

It's a variable that can be changed, but I suggest a 2-0-2-0 tempo or a 2-0-3-0 tempo to start with. These numbers mean that whenever the load is rising against gravity, allow 2 seconds for the movement to occur (the first 2), avoid pausing (the 0) and then take 2-3 seconds for the load to lower towards the floor, and repeat without pausing (the other 0).

This is a safe tempo because it avoids rapid, uncontrolled movements that may put unnecessary stress on the joints, muscles and connective tissue, but is also an effective tempo as the muscles have sufficient time under tension (TUT), particularly during the lowering phase when gravity can do the work for you!

Breathing

Breathing patterns can affect blood pressure and also the support your lumbar vertebrae get from intra-abdominal pressure.

To keep these optimal, aim to breathe continuously (avoid holding your breath) and ideally breathe out (exhale) when the load rises against gravity, and breathe in (inhale) when the load lowers towards the floor with gravity.

Chapter 11

The Essential Eight

The Essential Eight are the movement patterns that should create the foundation for all strength training after 50. They are the *fundamental* strength training exercises. Any other strength training movement patterns are not a necessity for maintaining a strong, healthy, well-functioning body in our later years.

The Essential Eight are as follows:

1. The Squat
2. The Hinge
3. The Step Up
4. The Horizontal Pull
5. The Vertical Pull
6. The Horizontal Push
7. The Vertical Push
8. The Carry

To support the exercise instructions and images within this section, I am providing you with exercise technique videos. See the webpage in the bonus material at the beginning of the book to gain access.

Let's look at each of *The Essential Eight*...

The Squat

The squat trains all the major muscle groups in the lower body; Quadriceps, Gluteus Maximus, Hamstrings, and Calf muscles.

In terms of movement, the squat is essential for human function. It's how we sit on and get up from a chair, the sofa, bed, and the toilet! It allows us to 'crouch down' (and back up) to pick things up off the floor, open low cupboards, and get in and out of cars.

The squat is a natural human movement, one that we can do from around 1 year of age. As years go by, the less we squat and the less capable of squatting we become! Hours of sitting cause muscles to tighten and/or weaken, as well as a reduction in joint mobility, muscular flexibility, and balance.

We can all still squat, but the coordination, efficiency, strength, endurance, and balance deteriorate throughout life unless we maintain our capabilities. If this continues to deteriorate, our chances of being able to perform this fundamental movement in our later years diminish, and subsequently, our quality of life becomes poorer.

In terms of an exercise, there are multiple variations of a squat, all of which target the same main working muscles; those that improve our ability to perform the activities of daily living outlined above.

When you think of the squat as an exercise, it may be a daunting prospect to have a barbell loaded with weight plates on your back while you attempt to perform your best effort of a squat. However, the Barbell Back Squat is just one variation of a squat.

I want this book to provide you with an effective strength training approach that is safe, simple and manageable. I will therefore provide you with enough squat variations, including progressions/regressions, to find the most suitable for you, dependent upon your capabilities, experience, confidence, and equipment available.

Chair Squat

Target Muscles: Quadriceps, Glutes, Hamstrings, Calves

Outline: It is the easiest version of a squat, so if you are new to exercise, or have not exercised for a long time, then I suggest you start with this version of the Squat. Aim to perfect the technique in the chair squat and be able to perform 15 repetitions comfortably before moving on to more challenging squat variations.

Equipment: Stable chair or bench.

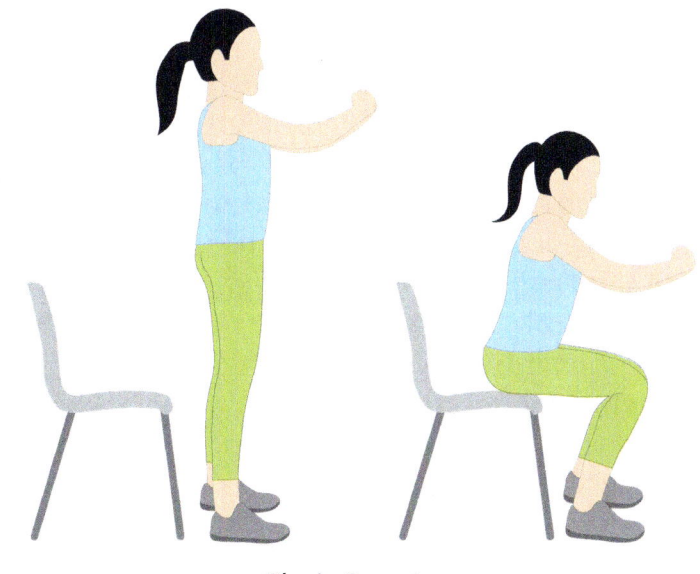

Chair Squats

Instructions:

1) Stand in front of your chair with your feet shoulder-width apart, toes pointing forward (or slightly outwards), arms in front of the chest for balance, shoulder blades back and down (chest open & shoulders relaxed), and core braced.

2) Start the movement by pushing the bum back and then bending the knees as if you are going to sit down. Keep weight distributed

evenly between the feet and maintain full contact between the feet and the floor.

3) Keep the chest lifted and core braced, breathing in on the way down.

4) Pause when your bum touches the chair.

5) Push your feet firmly into the ground and breathe out as you return to a standing position.

6) Finish standing tall with glutes fully contracting (glute squeeze).

Key Points:

- Keep three points of contact between your feet and the ground. One point is behind the big toe, one is behind the little toe, and one on the heel. Think of these three points as a tripod and keep them grounded at all times. Ensure weight stays distributed evenly. Always keep the heels grounded and avoid weight shifting into the balls of the feet.
- Keep a neutral curve in your spine. Achieve this by tilting the pelvis fully forwards, then backwards, then finding a midpoint with a slight inward curve of your lower back (before you start). Keep your core braced, chest open (& slightly lifted), and shoulders relaxed back and down.
- Breathe in on the way down, breathe out on the way up.
- At the bottom of the chair squat, aim for your torso to be at the same angle as your lower leg from a side view (use a mirror or record yourself).
- Ensure your knees track in line with your toes. Most faults result in the knees caving inwards; to prevent this, subtly screw your feet into the ground in an outwards direction and keep tension in your glutes throughout the move.

Bodyweight Squat

Target Muscles: Quadriceps, Glutes, Hamstrings, Calves

Outline: This is a little more challenging than chair squats. Ensure you can perform 15+ chair squats with good technique before moving on to this exercise. Again, make sure you can comfortably perform 15+ bodyweight squats with good technique before moving on to goblet squats.

Equipment: None.

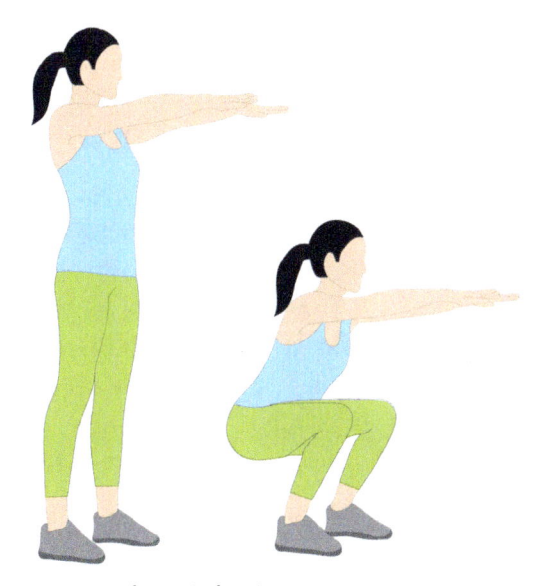

Bodyweight Squats

Instructions:

1) Stand with your feet shoulder-width apart, toes pointing forward (or slightly outwards), arms in front of the chest for balance, shoulder blades back and down (chest open & shoulders relaxed), and core braced.

2) Start the movement by pushing the bum back slightly and then bending the knees as if you are going to sit down. Keep weight distributed evenly between the feet and maintain full contact between the feet and the floor.

3) Keep the chest lifted and core braced, breathing in on the way down.

4) Aim to get your thighs parallel to the floor, or as low as possible without compromising technique.

5) Push your feet firmly into the ground and breathe out as you return to a standing position.

6) Finish standing tall with glutes fully contracting (glute squeeze).

Key Points:

- Keep three points of contact between your feet and the ground. One point is behind the big toe, one is behind the little toe, and one on the heel. Think of these three points as a tripod and keep them grounded at all times. Ensure weight stays distributed evenly. Always keep the heels grounded and avoid weight shifting into the balls of the feet.
- Keep a neutral curve in your spine. Achieve this by tilting the pelvis fully forwards, then backwards, then finding a midpoint with a slight inward curve of your lower back (before you start). Keep your core braced, chest open (& slightly lifted), and shoulders relaxed back and down.
- Breathe in on the way down, breathe out on the way up.
- At the bottom of the bodyweight squat, aim for your torso to be at the same angle as your lower leg, from a side view (use a mirror or record yourself).
- Your technique, as well as your mobility, will dictate the depth of your squat. Aim for thighs parallel to the floor, but go as low as possible without losing neutral spinal alignment. Torso angle similar to that of the lower leg, and ensure feet stay grounded, particularly the heels.

- Ensure your knees track in line with your toes. Most faults result in the knees caving inwards; to prevent this, subtly screw your feet into the ground in an outwards direction and keep tension in your glutes throughout the move.

Goblet Squat

Target Muscles: Quadriceps, Glutes, Hamstrings, Calves

Outline: This is more challenging than bodyweight squats and can vary in intensity depending on the weight you use. Ensure you can perform 15+ bodyweight squats with good technique before moving on to this exercise, and start with a relatively lightweight and progress appropriately. If you are comfortably performing 15 repetitions with a weight, it's time to progress the weight to make it a little more challenging.

Equipment: Dumbbell, Kettlebell, Sandball, Medicine Ball, or tin of beans!

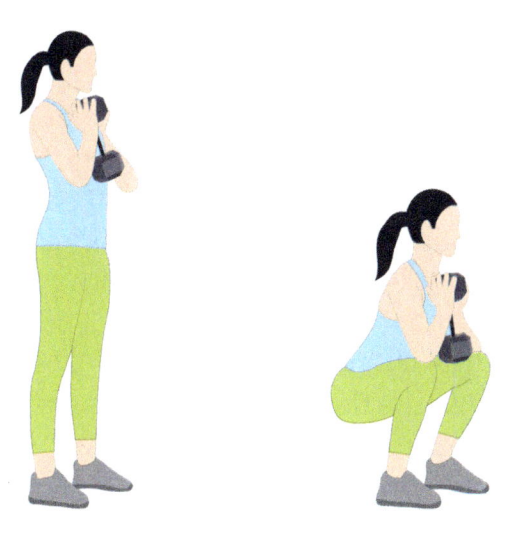

Goblet Squat

Instructions:

1) Stand with your feet shoulder-width apart, toes pointing slightly outwards, up to 30°. Hold your chosen weight close to your chest with your elbows under your wrists. Chest open, shoulders relaxed, and core braced.

2) Start the movement by pushing the bum back slightly and then bending the knees as if you are going to sit down. Keep weight distributed evenly between the feet and maintain full contact between the feet and the floor.

3) Keep the chest lifted and core braced, breathing in on the way down.

4) Aim to get your thighs parallel to the floor, or as low as possible without compromising technique.

5) Push your feet firmly into the ground and breathe out as you return to a standing position.

6) Finish standing tall with glutes fully contracting (glute squeeze).

Key Points:

- Keep three points of contact between your feet and the ground. One point is behind the big toe, one is behind the little toe, and one on the heel. Think of these three points as a tripod and keep them grounded at all times. Ensure weight stays distributed evenly. Always keep the heels grounded and avoid weight shifting into the balls of the feet.
- Keep a neutral curve in your spine. Achieve this by tilting the pelvis fully forwards, then backwards, then finding a midpoint with a slight inward curve of your lower back (before you start). Keep your core braced, chest open (& slightly lifted), and shoulders relaxed back and down.
- Breathe in on the way down, breathe out on the way up.
- Move your elbows away from your body as you descend, to keep them directly under your wrists.

- At the bottom of the goblet squat, aim for your torso to be at the same angle as your lower leg, from a side view (use a mirror or record yourself).
- Your technique, as well as your mobility, will dictate the depth of your squat. Aim for thighs parallel to the floor, but go as low as possible without losing neutral spinal alignment. Torso angle similar to that of the lower leg, and ensure feet stay grounded, particularly the heels.
- Ensure your knees track in line with your toes. Most faults result in the knees caving inwards; to prevent this, subtly screw your feet into the ground in an outwards direction and keep tension in your glutes throughout the move.

Sandbag/Powerbag Front Squat

Target Muscles: Quadriceps, Glutes, Hamstrings, Calves

Outline: This is more challenging than the other squat variations outlined above and can vary in intensity depending upon the weight you use. Ensure you can perform goblet squats with good technique before moving on to this exercise. Start with a relatively lightweight and progress appropriately. If you are comfortably performing 15 repetitions with a weight, it's time to progress the weight to make it a little more challenging.

Equipment: Powerbag or Sandbag.

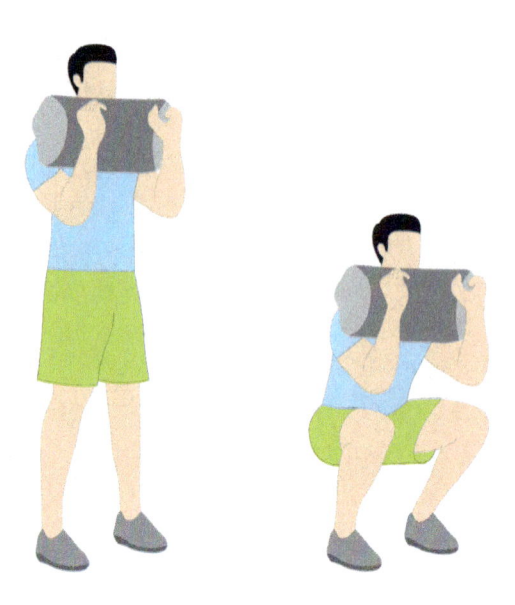

Powerbag Front Squat

Instructions:

1) Stand with your feet shoulder-width apart, toes pointing slightly outwards, up to 30°. Hold your chosen weight close to your chest with your elbows forward and powerboat/sandbag resting on the chest. Chest open, shoulders relaxed, and core braced.

2) Start the movement by pushing the bum back slightly and then bending the knees as if you are going to sit down. Keep weight distributed evenly between the feet and maintain full contact between the feet and the floor.

3) Keep the chest lifted and core braced, breathing in on the way down.

4) Aim to get your thighs parallel to the floor, or as low as possible without compromising technique.

5) Push your feet firmly into the ground and breathe out as you return to a standing position.

6) Finish standing tall with glutes fully contracted (glutes clenched!).

Key Points:

- Keep three points of contact between your feet and the ground. One point is behind the big toe, one is behind the little toe, and one on the heel. Think of these three points as a tripod and keep them grounded at all times. Ensure weight stays distributed evenly. Always keep the heels grounded and avoid weight shifting into the balls of the feet.
- Keep a neutral curve in your spine. Achieve this by tilting the pelvis fully forwards, then backwards, then finding a midpoint with a slight inward curve of your lower back (before you start). Keep your core braced, chest open (& slightly lifted), and shoulders relaxed back and down.
- Breathe in on the way down, breathe out on the way up.
- Keep your elbows pointing away from you in a forward direction.
- At the bottom of the front squat, aim for your torso to be at the same angle as your lower leg, from a side view (use a mirror or record yourself).
- Your technique, as well as your mobility, will dictate the depth of your squat. Aim for thighs parallel to the floor, but go as low as possible without losing neutral spinal alignment. Torso angle similar to that of the lower leg, and ensure feet stay grounded, particularly the heels.
- Ensure your knees track in line with your toes. Most faults result in the knees caving inwards; to prevent this, subtly screw your feet into the ground in an outwards direction and keep tension in your glutes throughout the move.

Additional versions of the Squat such as the Powerbag Back Squat and Barbell Back Squat can be seen in the relevant Exercise Technique Video (see webpage in bonus material).

The Hip Hinge

Exercises that involve the 'hip hinge' predominantly strengthen an area of the body known as the posterior chain.

The posterior chain comprises the Gluteus Maximus, Hamstrings, and Lumbar Extensors. These are the primary muscles required to extend the hips in movements that involve forward propulsion such as walking, running, climbing steps/stairs, as well as movements that involve lifting objects from the floor to a standing position. The posterior chain is considered to be the powerhouse of human movement.

The posterior chain also plays a significant role in stabilising the pelvis and maintaining optimal posture.

The Gluteus Maximus (Glute Max) is the largest muscle in the human body, therefore the importance of the hip hinge to keep this large muscle strong and functioning efficiently should not be underestimated.

It is extremely common for this important muscle to adapt negatively to the excessive time spent sitting down in our modern lives, whether it be at a desk, car, sofa, or chair.

When seated, we put the Glute Max into a stretched/lengthened position and over time, it will adapt to become both lengthened and weak/under-active. This, along with shortened/overactive opposing muscles (Hip Flexors), compromises pelvic and spinal posture, commonly leading to low back pain.

A strong and well-functioning posterior chain can counteract the negative impact of prolonged sitting and can prevent lower back pain.

As well as improving daily movement patterns, hip hinge exercises can improve pelvic/spinal posture, reducing the risk of associated low back pain.

Exercises that involve the hip hinge include the:

- Deadlift (various types)
- Kettlebell Swing
- Glute Bridge
- Hip Thrust

The following are my recommendations for performing hip hinge exercises after 50:

Kettlebell Deadlift

Target Muscles: Glutes and Hamstrings

Outline:

The Kettlebell Deadlift is one of the simplest and safest versions of a deadlift, but is also highly effective when performed with great technique and an appropriate weight. As well as strengthening the buttocks (glutes) and back of the thighs (hamstrings), there is also a small amount of work in the front of the thigh (quadriceps), and significant strengthening of the lower back and core.

The kettlebell deadlift is easier to master than using an Olympic barbell and is also more affordable and space-saving in a home environment. Kettlebells usually range from 4kg/9lb to 48kg/106lb, allowing a very manageable starting weight with plenty of room for progression.

Equipment: Kettlebell.

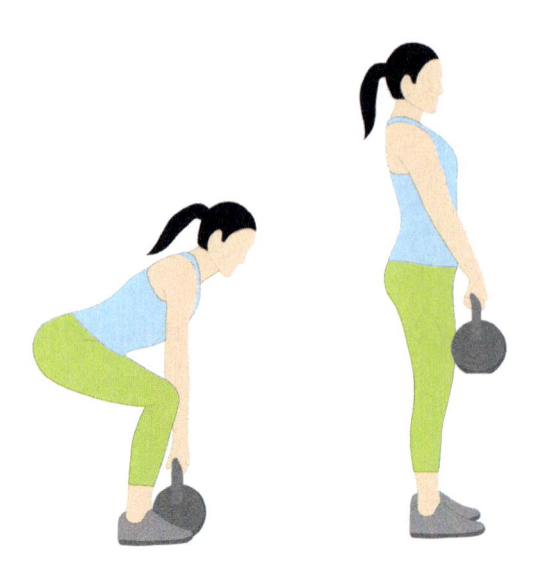

Kettlebell Deadlift

Instructions:

1) Stand with your feet shoulder-width apart, toes pointing slightly outwards, up to 30°, with the kettlebell centred between the balls of your feet.

2) Hinge your hips backwards, tipping from the hips with a slight knee bend until your torso reaches approximately 30° from the floor. Wrap both hands around the kettlebell handle. Before you lift, open up your chest, pull your shoulder blades back and down, brace your core, and tilt your head to keep the neck in line with the rest of the spine. Ensure your spine has and maintains natural curves.

3) Drive your feet into the ground lifting the kettlebell off the floor. Keep your arms straight and exhale as you rise.

4) Finish with the kettlebell resting in front of your body, glutes fully engaged (clench them!), core remaining engaged, chest open, shoulder blades back and down, looking straight ahead.

5) Hinge your hips backwards again, tipping from the hips with a slight knee bend until your torso reaches approximately 30° from the floor and the kettlebell touches down. Breathe in on the way down.

6) Repeat.

Key Points:

- Ensure the kettlebell is between your feet when you start, not out in front of you.
- Keep your feet fully grounded throughout.
- Keep a neutral curve in your spine. Achieve this by tilting the pelvis fully forwards, then backwards, then finding a midpoint with a slight inward curve of your lower back (before you start). Keep your core braced, chest open (& slightly lifted), and shoulder blades back and down.
- Breathe in on the way down, breathe out on the way up.
- Keep the kettlebell directly under your shoulders throughout.
- At the bottom of the deadlift, aim for approximately a 30° angle from the floor. Video yourself from the side and check.
- Ensure your knees only bend a small amount. The height of the hips should be approximately halfway between the knees and the shoulders at the bottom of the deadlift.

Suitcase Deadlift

Target Muscles: Glutes and Hamstrings

Outline: Although you can perform this exercise with two kettlebells, one in each hand, we are going to focus on the single-arm version. As the name suggests, this exercise is like lifting a suitcase from the floor to a standing position.

It predominantly utilizes the glutes and hamstrings on both sides of the body, but also adds a core strengthening element. With the weight only on one side, you will build strength in the core muscles that create (& prevent) sideways (lateral) stability of the spine.

To balance the work between the left and right sides of the body, the suitcase deadlift will need to be performed with the kettlebell in the left hand and in the right hand. Because of the load being off-centre, it is more challenging than the standard kettlebell deadlift, therefore, master the Kettlebell Deadlift before performing the Suitcase Deadlift.

Equipment: Kettlebell.

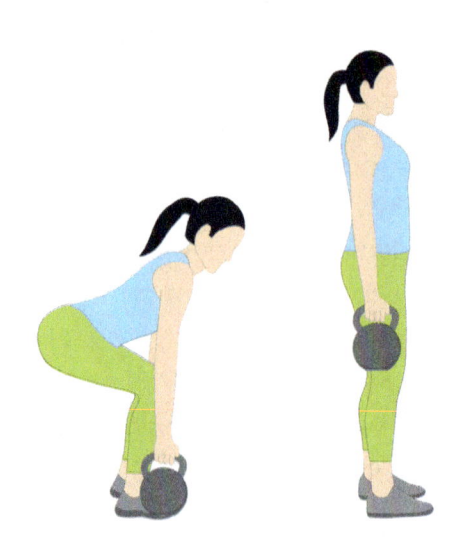

Suitcase Deadlift

Instructions:

1) Stand with your feet hip-shoulder width apart, toes pointing straight ahead or slightly outwards, with the kettlebell positioned to the outside of the ball of one foot.

2) Hinge your hips backwards, tipping from the hips with a slight knee bend until your torso reaches approximately 30° from the floor. Wrap one hand around the kettlebell handle.

3) Before you lift, open up your chest, square up your shoulders and pull your shoulder blades back and down, brace your core, and tilt your head to keep the neck in line with the rest of the spine. Ensure your spine has and maintains natural curves.

4) Drive your feet into the ground lifting the kettlebell off the floor. Keep your arms straight and exhale as you rise.

5) Finish with the kettlebell resting alongside your body, glutes fully engaged (clench them!), core remaining engaged, chest proud, shoulder blades back and down, looking straight ahead.

6) Hinge your hips backwards again, tipping from the hips with a slight knee bend until your torso reaches approximately 30° from the floor and the kettlebell touches down. Breathe in on the way down.

7) Repeat.

Key Points:

- Ensure the kettlebell is positioned *next* to your foot, not out in front of you.
- Keep your feet fully grounded throughout.
- Keep a neutral curve in your spine. Achieve this by tilting the pelvis fully forwards, then backwards, then finding a midpoint with a slight inward curve of your lower back (before you start). Keep your core braced, chest open (& slightly lifted), and shoulder blades back and down.
- Breathe in on the way down, breathe out on the way up.
- Keep the kettlebell directly under your shoulders (from a side view) throughout.
- At the bottom of the deadlift, aim for approximately a 30° angle from the floor. Video yourself from the side and check.

- Ensure your knees only bend a small amount. The height of the hips should be approximately halfway between the knees and the shoulders at the bottom of the deadlift.

Single-Leg Deadlift

Target Muscles: Glutes and Hamstrings

Outline: The Single-Leg Deadlift is the most technical and challenging of the three types of Deadlift we are covering. It works one side of the body at a time, known as a unilateral exercise.

As well as strengthening the glutes and hamstrings, its benefits include improving any imbalances between the muscles on the left and right side of the body, improving balance which is vital as we get older, and challenging the core muscles to prevent any unwanted rotation through the trunk.

I would suggest mastering the Kettlebell Deadlift and Suitcase Deadlift before attempting the Single-Leg Deadlift and starting with no weight or a very lightweight.

Equipment: Kettlebell or Dumbbell.

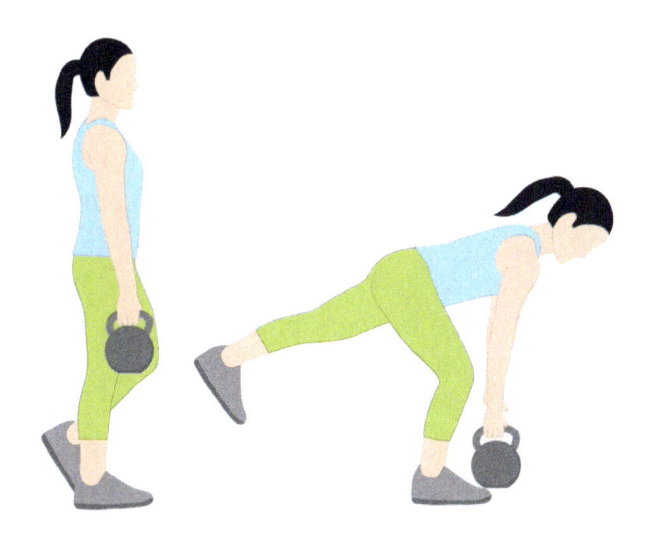

Single-Leg Deadlift

Instructions:

1) Hold a kettlebell in your right hand and rest it on your thigh. Set your shoulder blades back and down, brace your core, and look straight ahead. Lift your left foot slightly off the ground and ensure you have a slight bend in your right knee.

2) Hinge your hips backwards along with your left leg, tipping from the hips with a slight bend in the right knee until your torso reaches approximately 30° from the floor. Allow the kettlebell to hang under the right shoulder and keep your neck in line with the rest of the spine. Ensure your spine maintains its natural curves. Inhale as you descend.

3) Drive your right foot into the ground, returning the body to its upright position again. Exhale as you rise.

4) Finish in the start position, right glute fully engaged (clench it!), core remaining engaged, chest proud, shoulder blades back and down, looking straight ahead.

5) Repeat for the desired number of repetitions and then change legs.

Key Points:

- Keep the foot on the floor fully grounded throughout.
- Keep a neutral curve in your spine. Achieve this by tilting the pelvis fully forwards, then backwards, then finding a midpoint with a slight inward curve of your lower back (before you start). Keep your core braced, chest open (& slightly lifted), and shoulder blades back and down.
- Breathe in on the way down, breathe out on the way up.
- Keep the kettlebell directly under your shoulder throughout.
- At the bottom of the Single-Leg Deadlift, aim for approximately a 30° angle from the floor, shoulders higher than hips. Video yourself from the side and check.
- Ensure your knees only bend a small amount. The hips should remain positioned well above the knees.

2-Arm Kettlebell Swing

Target Muscles: Glutes and Hamstrings

Outline: The 2-Arm Kettlebell Swing is one of the most fundamental kettlebell-specific exercises and is the most dynamic of the exercises that we are going to look at. It utilizes the posterior chain muscles in a relatively dynamic and explosive manner, giving it a slightly steeper learning curve than the other hip hinge exercises.

As well as improving strength and power in the posterior chain, it is a great exercise for building a bulletproof core, increasing grip and wrist strength, boosting aerobic capacity, reducing lower back pain (if performed correctly), and burning fat.

Because of the range of kettlebell weights available, it is advisable to start with a lightweight to focus on the technique and progress slowly. Once ready to progress, you can either increase the weight of the kettlebell or perform one of the progressions in the hip hinge technique video (see bonus material).

As this is a relatively dynamic, fast-moving exercise, I highly recommend accessing the technique videos to complement the instructions and image below.

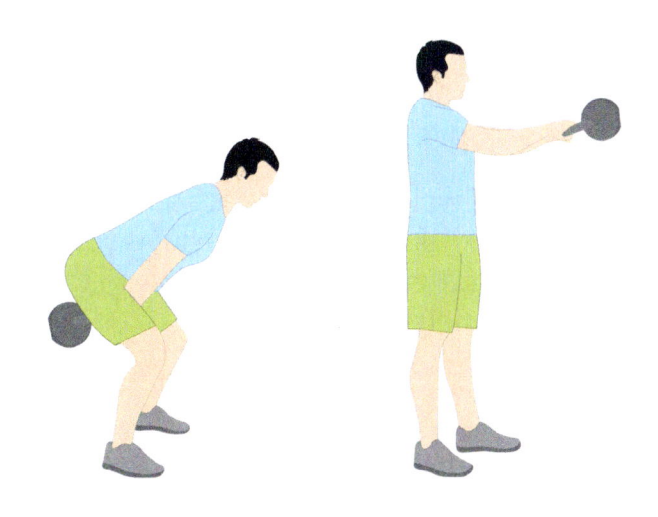

Equipment: Kettlebell.

Kettlebell Swing

Instructions:

1) Pick up the kettlebell in the same way you did during the kettlebell deadlift. Stand with your feet slightly wider than shoulder-width, toes pointing outwards, approximately 30°. Set your shoulder blades back and down, chest lifted, brace your core, and look straight ahead.

2) From the start position, start the swing by shifting the hips back slightly and immediately thrusting them forwards. Allow the kettlebell to swing between the thighs whilst pushing the hips

back, with a slight bend of the knees until your torso reaches approximately 30° from the floor. Ensure your spine maintains natural curves, including the neck.

3) Perform a 'hip snap' by dynamically thrusting the hips in a forward direction, allowing the kettlebell to 'swing' through to shoulder height. Keep your arms almost straight with a slight bend at the elbow, shoulder blades remain back and down and exhale on the way through to the top.

4) Engage the glutes in full extension of the hips, with the base of the KB facing away from the body. Keep the core braced to maintain neutral curves in the spine and to avoid arching the lower back. Look straight ahead, over the top of the kettlebell.

5) After a moment of weightlessness at shoulder height, let gravity allow the kettlebell to drop naturally. Hinge your hips backwards again, allowing the kettlebell to swing between the thighs, with the handles above knee height.

6) Repeat the 'hip snap' for the next repetition and continue this sequence until the set is complete.

Key Points:

- This is a relatively fast, dynamic movement rather than slow and steady.
- Keep your feet fully grounded throughout, outside shoulder width to allow the kettlebell to pass through the thighs.
- Keep a neutral curve in your spine. Achieve this by tilting the pelvis fully forwards, then backwards, then finding a midpoint with a slight inward curve of your lower back (before you start). Keep your core braced, chest proud (slightly lifted), and shoulders relaxed back and down.
- Breathe in on the way down, breathe out on the way up.
- When the kettlebell passes between the legs, ensure the handle stays above your knee height, otherwise, it will cause excessive forces on the lower back. To achieve this, let the

kettlebell drop from shoulder height <u>before</u> you tip from your hips.
- Use the 'hip snap' to swing the kettlebell through to shoulder height. Avoid lifting with your shoulder muscles. The bottom of the kettlebell should face away from you when at shoulder height.
- At the bottom of the swing, aim for your torso to be approximately 30° angle from the floor. Video yourself from the side and check.
- Ensure your knees only bend a small amount to avoid squatting, and keep your knees pushed out in line with your toes.

Glute Bridge

Target Muscle: Gluteus Maximus

Outline: The Glute Bridge is a must-do exercise for targeting the Glute Max as the primary working muscle, with minimal input from secondary muscles. This is vitally important if your glutes have become weak and under-active because of inactivity and prolonged sitting through desk-bound work, driving, watching tv, etc.

Weak and under-active glutes, along with tight and overactive opposing muscles, can cause postural problems that can lead to lower back pain and a lack of functional capabilities. We cover this in more detail in book five of the *Simple Fitness After 50* Series.

The Glute Bridge is relatively easy to perform and can be done with no equipment. There are several variations with room for progression by adding load to the front of the hips, and by moving on to Hip Thrusts (covered next).

Equipment: Mat.

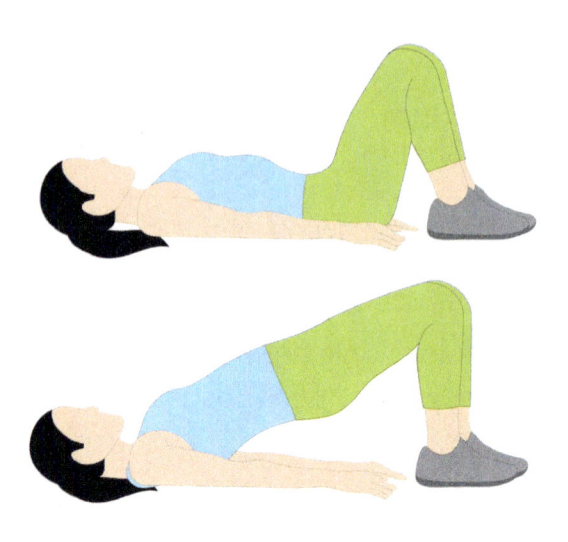

Glute Bridge

Instructions:

1) Lay on the floor, or a mat, with your arms resting on the floor alongside your body. Bend the knees until your feet are flat on the floor and your heels are close to your fingertips. Feet should be hip-shoulder width apart with and straight or slightly turned out. Brace the core before commencing.

2) Push through your heels, lifting your hips until you have a straight line from your shoulders, through your hips, to your knees. Squeeze your glutes together at the top whilst tilting your pelvis posteriorly (so the front of your pelvis moves towards your ribs), and exhale. Drive your knees out slightly to ensure they stay aligned between your hips and toes.

3) Lower your hips under control, inhaling as you descend, until you feel the floor and drive back up again.

4) If you feel the work in the front of the thighs (quads), try performing the exercise with your feet slightly further away

from your body. If you feel the work in the back of the thighs (hamstrings), try performing the exercise with your feet slightly closer to the body. Find the position that maximizes the work in the glutes.

5) Experiment with your foot width. Try it with the feet hip-width and the toes pointing forwards, then try with the feet shoulder-width and the toes turned out slightly. Find the spot that maximizes the work in your glutes. The wider the feet go, the more you will need to turn your toes out.

Key Points:

- Experiment with foot positioning to optimize the glute engagement.
- Keep your feet fully grounded, or if you have a tendency to push through the balls of your feet or your toes, try bringing the toes off the ground towards your shins, leaving only your heels on the ground
- To further engage the glutes, and avoid arching the lower back, tilt the pelvis backwards (posteriorly) at the top of the movement. Bring the front of the pelvis towards your ribs.
- Aim to keep the ribs low rather than pushing them upwards towards the top of the movement.
- Breathe in on the way down, breathe out on the way up.
- An alternative arm position is to bend the elbows until your forearms are vertical, wrists over elbows, and clench your fists. Use whichever is most comfortable for you.

Weighted Hip Thrusts

Target Muscle: Gluteus Maximus

Outline: The Hip Thrust is like the Glute Bridge, but performed with the upper back raised on a bench (or similar). It is a little harder to master than the Glute Bridge, but is still a relatively simple exercise to learn.

The rewards for the higher difficulty, compared to the Glute Bridge, are; you can perform the Hip Thrust through a greater range of motion (ROM) thus providing more time under tension, lift heavier loads creating greater tension on the glutes, and the body position lends itself to the more ergonomic lifting of weights.

It also has all the benefits discussed under the Glute Bridge, albeit with more difficulty, but with greater potential. It requires some additional equipment, so isn't as accessible as the Glute Bridge. I would suggest mastering the Glute Bridge prior to progressing to Hip Thrusts.

Equipment: Bench or Hip Thruster Machine, Sandbag, Barbell, or Dumbbells.

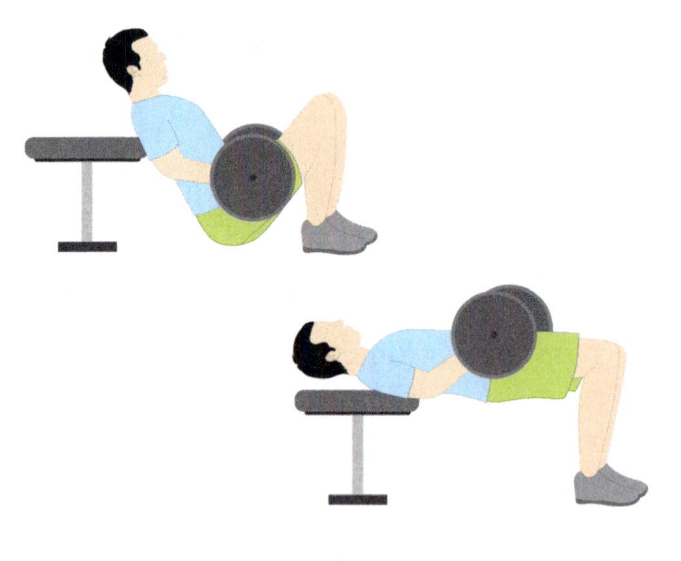

Hip Thrusts

Instructions:

1) Sit on the floor with a stable bench (or similar), which is approximately 14"/35cm high, behind you. If using weight, position it just above your pubic bone, and use cushioning if necessary. Rest

your upper back, just under your shoulder blades, onto the edge of the bench. Bend the knees, bringing the heels closer to the body. You'll need to check the foot positioning when you get to the top of the movement; aim for your lower leg to be approximately vertical. Hold your chosen weight with your hands and rest your upper arms on the edge of the bench. Brace your core. When you are set up correctly, your glutes are likely to be off the ground.

2) Push through your heels, lifting your hips until you have a straight line from your shoulders, through your hips, to your knees. Squeeze your glutes together at the top whilst tilting your pelvis posteriorly (so the front of your pelvis moves towards your ribs), and exhale. Drive your knees out slightly to ensure they stay aligned between your hips and toes. Tuck your chin towards your chest as you rise, so you are looking ahead (if this is uncomfortable, look up instead.

3) Lower your hips under control, inhaling as you descend, until you return to your start position, and drive back up again.

4) If you feel the work in the front of the thighs (quads), try performing the exercise with your feet slightly further away from your body. If you feel the work in the back of the thighs (hamstrings), try performing the exercise with your feet slightly closer to the body. Find the position that maximizes the work in the glutes.

5) Experiment with your foot width. Try it with the feet hip-width and the toes pointing forwards, then try with the feet shoulder-width and the toes turned out slightly. Find the spot that maximizes the work in your glutes. The wider the feet go, the more you will need to turn your toes out.

Key Points:

- Experiment with foot positioning to optimize the glute engagement.
- Keep your feet fully grounded, or if you have a tendency to push through the balls of your feet or your toes, try bringing the

toes off the ground towards your shins, leaving only your heels on the ground
- To further engage the glutes, and avoid arching the lower back, tilt the pelvis backwards (posteriorly) at the top of the movement. Bring the front of the pelvis towards your ribs.
- Aim to keep the ribs low rather than pushing them upwards towards the top of the movement. Aim for a neutral spine at the bottom and the posterior pelvic tilt at the top; initiate movement from below your breastbone (sternum).
- Breathe in on the way down, breathe out on the way up.
- If you're performing a Bodyweight Hip Thrust, clench your fists and bend the elbows until your knuckles point upwards. Press the upper arms into the bench.

The Step Up

Step Ups train all the major muscle groups in the lower body; Quadriceps, Gluteus Maximus, Hamstrings, and Calf muscles. These are essentially the same muscles as the squat, but via a different movement pattern.

So, why complete Step Ups in addition to the squat? Despite the two exercises utilizing the same muscles, they are different in terms of movement pattern and functionality. Step Ups are one of the most underrated exercises for many people, but particularly for those over 50.

Step Ups have three key features that make them stand out:

1. They are one of the most simple exercises to perform, with a very low risk of injury.
2. They are unilateral, which means you work one leg independently of the other leg, ensuring both legs work equally within the exercise and aiding in correcting any differences between the left and right leg.

3. They are very functional, meaning the movement pattern is one that is required regularly in everyday life. Think about how often you have to use stairs in a house/home/shops, use steps in an outdoor environment, walk uphill, as well as climbing over objects and using ladders.

We can easily perform Step Ups at the gym, at home, and/or outdoors, using a varied form of load including your body weight, barbell, dumbbells, kettlebells, sandbags, or powerbags.

As well as varying the type of equipment used, we will also cover a variety of types of Step Up including; Bodyweight Step Ups, Weighted Step Ups, Lateral Step Ups, and Lateral Step Downs.

Bodyweight Step Ups

Target Muscles: Quadriceps, Glutes, Hamstrings, Calves

Outline: This is the easiest version of the Step Up, therefore a great starting point for this exercise. You can progress this exercise by increasing the height of the step; ideally, you want to be using a step with a height that causes your knee to be at, or slightly above, hip height when your foot is resting on top. Start lower than this and progress once you can comfortably perform 12+ repetitions on each leg. If you are comfortably performing 12+ reps/leg at the ideal step height, progress to Weighted Step Ups.

Equipment: Step.

Bodyweight Step Ups

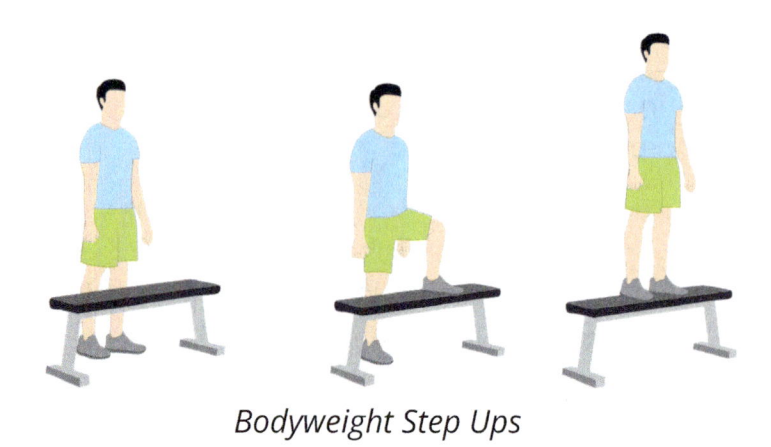

Instructions:

1) Stand with a step positioned in front of you, adjusted to your chosen height. Have your feet hip-width apart, toes pointing forward, arms by your side, shoulder blades back and down (chest open & shoulders relaxed), and core braced.

2) Place your left foot firmly onto the step and position the knee over the top of the toes (in front of the ankle). Drive through that foot, raising your body upwards and place the right foot on the step, maintaining the hip-width stance. Fully extend the hips and engage the glutes whilst keeping the core braced (to keep a neutral spinal alignment). Exhale as you rise to the top and look straight ahead.

3) Step down, under control, with your left leg and then the right, back to the start position. Inhale as you descend.

4) You can either alternate until you have achieved the desired repetitions on both legs, or repeat on the same leg until you have reached the desired repetitions, and then swap. If repeating on 1 leg, follow the pattern: LRLR, LRLR.... If alternating legs, follow the pattern: LRLR, RLRL, LRLR, RLRL...

Key Points:

- Keep a hip-width stance regardless of whether your feet are on the floor or the step.
- Keep a neutral curve in your spine. Achieve this by tilting the pelvis fully forwards, then backwards, then finding a midpoint with a slight inward curve of your lower back (before you start). Keep your core braced, chest proud (slightly lifted), and shoulders relaxed back and down.
- Breathe in on the way down, breathe out on the way up.
- Let your arms do their natural movement as you step up and down; this will help to maintain balance.
- Push up onto the step through a fully grounded front foot; heels down.

Dumbbell/Kettlebell Step Ups

Target Muscles: Quadriceps, Glutes, Hamstrings, Calves

Outline: The Dumbbell, or Kettlebell, Step Up is the weighted version of this exercise that we are going to look at. There are other weighted versions, but we are going to focus on using dumbbells or kettlebells as the next progression from Bodyweight Step Ups. Ensure you have mastered the bodyweight step up and can perform 12+ repetitions on each leg, at the ideal step height, before attempting this weighted version. When adding weight, lower the step temporarily while you adapt to the increased challenge, then focus on increasing the step height to its optimum before advancing with more weight.

Equipment: Step and either dumbbells or kettlebells.

Kettlebell Step Ups

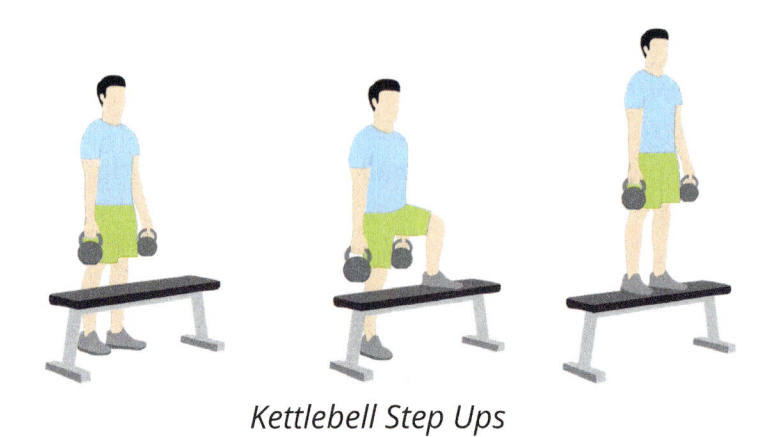

Instructions:

1) Stand with a step positioned in front of you, adjusted to your chosen height. Have your feet hip-width apart, toes pointing forward, arms by your side with dumbbells or kettlebells in your hands, shoulder blades back and down (chest open & shoulders relaxed), and core braced.

2) Place your left foot firmly onto the step and position the knee over the top of the toes (in front of the ankle). Drive through that foot, raising your body upwards and place the right foot on the step, maintaining the hip-width stance. Fully extend the hips and engage the glutes whilst keeping the core braced (to keep a neutral spinal alignment). Exhale as you rise to the top and look straight ahead.

3) Step down, under control, with your left leg and then the right, back to the start position. Inhale as you descend.

4) You can either alternate until you have achieved the desired repetitions on both legs, or repeat on the same leg until you have reached the desired repetitions, and then swap. If repeating on 1 leg, follow the pattern: LRLR, LRLR.... If alternating legs, follow the pattern: LRLR, RLRL, LRLR, RLRL...

Key Points:

- Keep a hip-width stance regardless of whether your feet are on the floor or the step.
- Keep a neutral curve in your spine. Achieve this by tilting the pelvis fully forwards, then backwards, then finding a midpoint with a slight inward curve of your lower back (before you start). Keep your core braced, chest proud (slightly lifted), and shoulders relaxed back and down.
- Breathe in on the way down, breathe out on the way up.
- Try to keep your arms by your sides, below the shoulders, throughout the exercise.
- Push up onto the step through a fully grounded front foot; heels down.

Lateral Step Ups (Bodyweight or Weighted)

Target Muscles: Quadriceps, Glutes, Hamstrings, Calves

Outline: Lateral Step Ups are slightly more challenging than conventional Step Ups; we are going to add in a balance element by keeping the non-working leg elevated rather than placing it on the step.

You can progress this exercise by increasing the height of the step; ideally, you want to be using a step with a height that causes your knee to be at, or slightly above, hip height when your foot is resting on top. Start lower than this and progress once you can comfortably perform 12+ repetitions on each leg. If you are comfortably performing 12+ reps/leg at the ideal step height, with good balance and stability, progress to weighted Lateral Step Ups.

Equipment: Step (and dumbbells or kettlebells, if weighted).

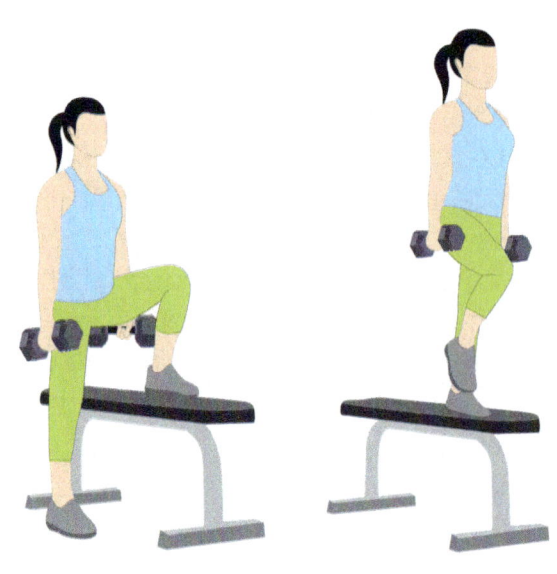

Lateral Step Ups

Instructions:

1) Stand with a step positioned to the side of you, adjusted to your chosen height. Have your feet hip-width apart, toes pointing forward, arms by your side, shoulder blades back and down (chest open & shoulders relaxed), and core braced. Hold dumbbells or kettlebells in your hands, if performing the weighted version.

2) Place the foot that's closest to the step firmly on top and position the knee over the top of the toes (in front of the ankle). Drive through that foot, raising your body upwards, keeping the opposing foot suspended in the air, knee slightly bent. Fully extend the hip on the working leg and engage the glutes whilst keeping the core braced (to keep a neutral spinal alignment). Exhale as you rise to the top and look straight ahead.

3) Step down, under control, until your non-working foot returns to the floor, back to the start position. Inhale as you descend.

4) Repeat on the same leg for the desired number of repetitions, ensuring you push through the foot on the step, not the one on the floor.

5) Change sides and repeat on the opposite leg.

Key Points:

- Keep the effort in the working leg and avoid pushing off through the non-working leg.
- Keep a neutral curve in your spine. Achieve this by tilting the pelvis fully forwards, then backwards, then finding a midpoint with a slight inward curve of your lower back (before you start). Keep your core braced, chest proud (slightly lifted), and shoulders relaxed back and down.
- Breathe in on the way down, breathe out on the way up.
- If performing the bodyweight version, let your arms do their natural movement as you step up and down; this will help to maintain balance. If using weights, try to keep them by the side of the body, below the shoulders.
- Push up onto the step through a fully grounded foot; heels down.

Lateral Step Downs

Target Muscles: Quadriceps, Glutes, Hamstrings, Calves

Outline: Lateral Step Downs are more challenging than Lateral Step Ups as they maintain tension in the muscles throughout the movement, and focus heavily on the descent during which the muscles lengthen under load (eccentric contractions) causing increased micro-tears in the muscles. This causes an increased need for recovery, may cause greater post-exercise soreness, and requires more muscle repair and rebuilding.

However, it can also produce significant increases in strength as well as control and coordination because of the emphasis on the deceleration of the downward phase of the exercise. It also aids balance, as we have minimal contact between the non-working foot and the floor, or step.

You can progress this exercise by increasing the height of the step; ideally, you want to be using a step with a height that causes your knee to be at hip height when your foot is resting on top. This is quite challenging in this exercise, so start much lower than this and progress once you can comfortably perform 10+ repetitions on each leg. If you are comfortable performing 10+ reps/leg at the ideal step height, with good balance and stability, progress to Weighted Lateral Step Downs.

Equipment: Step.

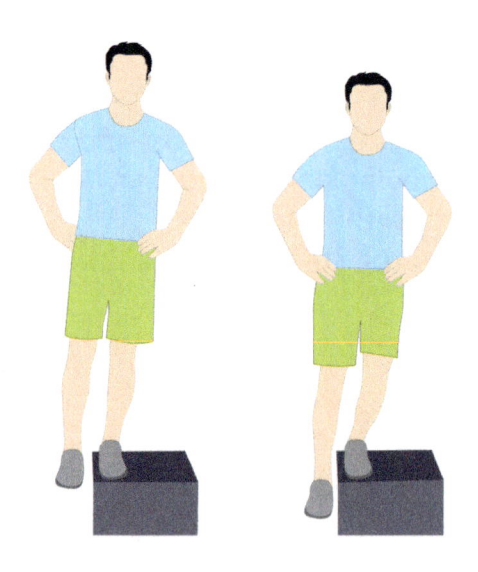

Lateral Step Downs

Instructions:

1) Stand with a step positioned to the side of you, adjusted to your chosen height. Stand on the step with one foot, with the other suspended over the edge of the step. Place your hands on your hips, or hold them out for balance. Toes pointing forward, shoulder

blades back and down (chest open & shoulders relaxed), and core braced. Hold dumbbells or kettlebells in your hands, if performing the weighted version.

2) Hinge your hips back and bend the knee of the working leg, lowering yourself slowly and under control until your non-working foot touches the ground. Keep the working muscles under tension by keeping your weight in your working leg, and just touching the ground with the non-working foot. Inhale as you descend.

3) Drive through your top foot to return to the start position, fully extending the hip and engaging the glutes. Keep the non-working leg suspended; try to avoid resting it on the step, if possible. Exhale as you rise.

4) Repeat on the same leg for the desired number of repetitions, ensuring you push through the foot on the step, not the one on the floor.

5) Change sides and repeat on the opposite leg.

Key Points:

- Keep the effort in the working leg and avoid pushing off through the non-working leg.
- Descend slowly, aiming for around 3 seconds on the way down.
- Ascend quicker, aiming for around 1 second on the way up.
- Keep a neutral curve in your spine. Achieve this by tilting the pelvis fully forwards, then backwards, then finding a midpoint with a slight inward curve of your lower back (before you start). Keep your core braced, chest proud (slightly lifted), and shoulders relaxed back and down.
- Breathe in on the way down, breathe out on the way up.
- If performing the bodyweight version, let your arms do their natural movement as you step up and down; this will help to maintain balance. If using weights, try to keep them by the side of the body, below the shoulders.

- Push up onto the step through a fully grounded foot; heels down (the foot on the step).

The 'Pull'

An exercise must meet all the following criteria to be categorized as a 'pull':

- Upper body movement
- Compound (2 or more moving joints)
- Involve pulling a load towards the upper body, or the upper body moving toward a fixed object during the pull

Pull exercises predominantly utilize the muscles of the back (Latissimus Dorsi, Trapezius, Rhomboids), back of the shoulders (Posterior/Rear Deltoids), and front of the arms (Biceps). They also utilize the muscles of the forearm to grip/hold the equipment being used.

As well as contributing towards overall upper body strength, the *pull* group of exercises play an important role in daily life, including those of later years, by improving our ability to lift objects with the upper body, pull open heavy doors, carry objects that require grip strength such as shopping bags, and helping to maintain a desirable upper body posture.

Upper body posture is negatively affected by modern-day living... using a computer at a desk, using smartphones, driving cars, and children (or adults) playing video games on consoles. Pull exercises help to recruit muscles that become weak/under-active in the most common upper body postural distortions, making them an integral part of any strength training program.

I have separated the pull into two separate exercise categories: *the horizontal pull* and *the vertical pull*. This helps to work the muscles through varied planes of motion (direction of movement), involves slightly different primary muscle groups, changes the range of motion a muscle works through and creates a more desirable muscle balance.

Putting the pull exercises into two separate categories also ensures you are not over-training one type of pull and under-training the other type of pull, and makes sure you are training these muscles in a way that they may be required in your everyday movement patterns.

The Horizontal Pull

A horizontal pull involves pulling a weight from in front of your body, towards you, or pulling your body towards an object (e.g. a bar) in front of your body.

Examples of a horizontal pull include; Seated Row, Standing Row, Bent Over Row, Single Arm Row, and Inverted Row.

Seated Band Rows

Target Muscles: Latissimus Dorsi, Posterior Deltoid, Mid & Lower Trapezius, Rhomboids, Biceps

Outline: This is a great starting point to increase strength in the back and bicep muscles. It is safe, simple and effective. Minimal and affordable equipment is required, meaning we can do it at home or at the gym.

Resistance bands come in various levels of resistance, allowing room to start easy and progress when required. Another way of progressing with resistance bands is to increase the stretch on the band before starting the exercise by positioning yourself further from the anchor point.

Aim to progress the resistance, or the exercise, when you can perform 15+ seated band rows with excellent technique.

Equipment: Chair or bench, resistance band, and something sturdy to provide an anchor for the band.

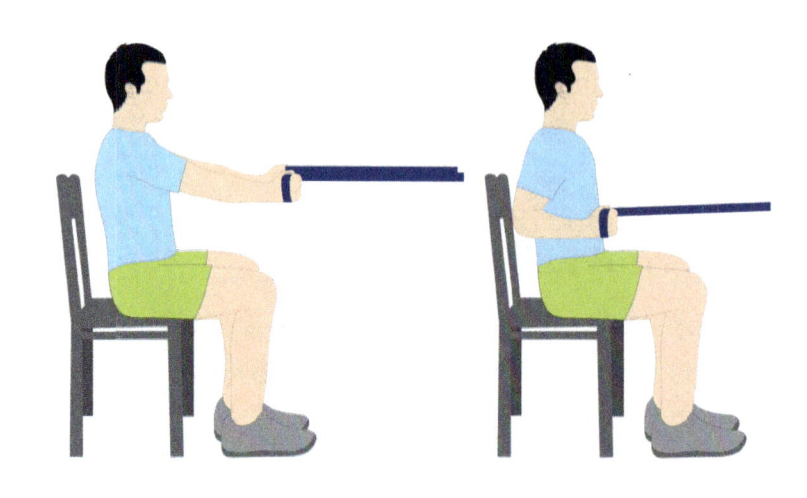

Seated Band Row

Instructions:

1) Attach two resistance bands to a sturdy object as an anchor point, around elbow height whilst seated. Sit on a chair or bench, facing the anchor point. Hold a band in each hand and ensure there is a slight stretch in the bands when the arms are outstretched. Set your feet shoulder-width with the ankles under the knees. Look straight ahead, roll the shoulders back and down and brace the core, creating a neutral spine.

2) Keeping your torso still, pull both elbows backwards brushing the side of the body, and keep the forearms parallel to the floor. Squeeze your shoulder blades together at the end of the movement. Exhale as you pull.

3) Reverse the movement until your arms are straight, but keep the tension between your shoulder blades. Inhale as you lengthen the arms.

4) Aim for around 2 seconds in (concentric phase) and 2 seconds out (eccentric phase).

5) Repeat for the desired number of repetitions before leaning forward to create slack in the band before you let go!

Key Points:

- The set-up will dictate the quality of the exercise, so follow step 1 above carefully.
- Keep a neutral curve in your spine. Achieve this by tilting the pelvis fully forwards, then backwards, then finding a midpoint with a slight inward curve of your lower back (before you start). Keep your core braced, chest open (& slightly lifted), and shoulders relaxed back and down.
- Breathe out as you pull, breathe in as you release.
- Keep your torso still and avoid leaning back or arching your back.
- Consciously bring your shoulder blades together (and down) at the end of the pull.
- Your forearms should stay parallel to the floor and in line with the bands (if you have set them up at the optimum height).

Standing One-Arm Band Row

Target Muscles: Latissimus Dorsi, Posterior Deltoid, Mid & Lower Trapezius, Rhomboids, Biceps, Core

Outline: This exercise places a couple of additional challenges on the body when compared to the seated band row, but is also relatively simple to perform and can be performed with a light resistance band before progressing to a higher intensity.

The first additional challenge comes from standing (vs. sitting), which creates a demand on the lower body to fixate and remain stabilized throughout the movement. The second additional challenge comes from performing the exercise with one arm (unilateral) as opposed to two arms simultaneously (bilateral). This helps you to focus on each arm individually, preventing you from dominating the exercise with your strongest side and also engages your core muscles to prevent unwanted rotation through the spine.

As with the Seated Band Row, you can progress the exercise by using a band with more resistance, or to a lesser extent, by increasing the stretch on the band before starting the exercise.

Aim to progress the resistance, or the exercise, when you can perform 15+ seated band rows with excellent technique.

Equipment: Resistance band, and something sturdy to provide an anchor for the band.

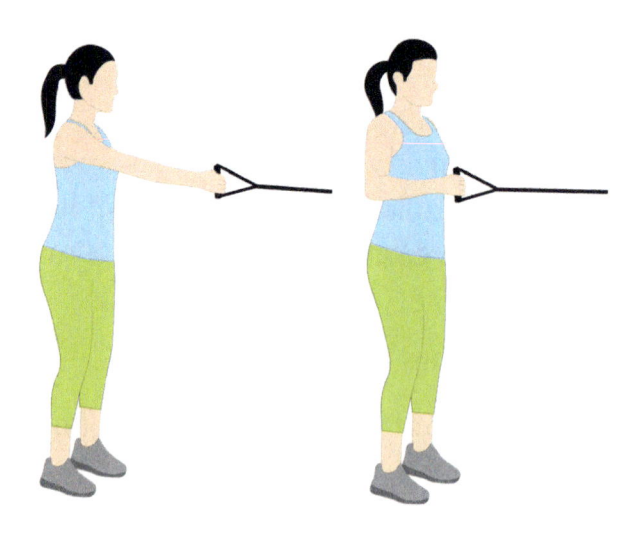

Standing One-Arm Band Row

Instructions:

1) Attach one resistance band to a sturdy object as an anchor point, around elbow height whilst standing. Face the anchor point, hold the band in one hand and ensure there is a slight stretch in the band when the arm is outstretched. Set your feet shoulder-width apart. If preferred, split your stance so the left foot is forward when the band is in the right hand, and vice versa.

2) Look straight ahead, roll the shoulders back and down and brace the core, creating a neutral spine. Unlock the knees slightly.

3) Keeping your torso still, pull the elbow backwards brushing the side of the body, and keep the forearm parallel to the floor. Squeeze your shoulder blades together at the end of the movement. Exhale as you pull.

4) Reverse the movement until your arm is straight, but keep the tension between your shoulder blades. Inhale as you lengthen the arms.

5) Aim for around 2 seconds in (concentric phase) and 2 seconds out (eccentric phase).

6) Repeat for the desired number of repetitions before switching to the other arm.

Key Points:

- The set-up will dictate the quality of the exercise, so follow step 1 above carefully.
- Keep a neutral curve in your spine. Achieve this by tilting the pelvis fully forwards, then backwards, then finding a midpoint with a slight inward curve of your lower back (before you start). Keep your core braced, chest open (& slightly lifted), and shoulders relaxed back and down.
- Breathe out as you pull, breathe in as you release.
- Keep your torso still and avoid twisting or arching your back.

- Consciously bring your shoulder blade back (and down) at the end of the pull.
- Your forearm should stay parallel to the floor and in line with the band (if you have set it up at the optimum height).

Bent-Over Row (Kettlebell or Dumbbell)

Target Muscles: Latissimus Dorsi, Posterior Deltoid, Mid & Lower Trapezius, Rhomboids, Biceps

Outline: The Bent-Over Row is a more advanced exercise than the previous horizontal pulls we have looked at. Despite the weights moving vertically, we consider the Bent-Over Row to be a horizontal pull because of the movement being perpendicular to the torso (you pull from in front of your torso because of the bent-over position).

As well as being a great exercise to strengthen the back and bicep muscles, it also requires the engagement of the core muscles and the lumbar extensors (the muscles in the lower back). This can be seen as a positive, but can also be a limiting factor of the exercise.

If being in the 'bent over' position causes excess stress or discomfort in the lower back and affects your ability to perform this exercise, then I suggest you leave this exercise for now. You can always return to it when you have gained more core strength (see *Simple Fitness After 50 – Book Two*).

Choose lightweight dumbbells or kettlebells for your first attempt and only progress the load when you can comfortably perform 15+ repetitions with great technique.

Equipment: Dumbbells or Kettlebells.

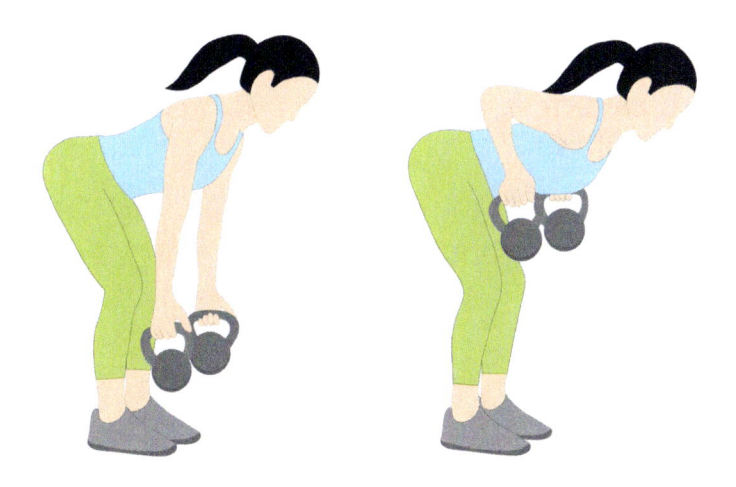

Kettlebell Bent-Over Row

Instructions:

1) Deadlift the dumbbells or kettlebells off the floor. If your back rounds/bends when picking up the weights, go down on one knee to pick them up.

2) Set the feet hip-width apart, roll the shoulder blades back and down, brace the core, and tip from the hip until your torso reaches 30-40° from the floor. Ensure you maintain neutral curves in your spine (video from the side and check, or use a mirror). Allow the weights to hang under your mid-sternum (breastbone). Keep your neck in line with the rest of the spine with your chin tucked slightly.

3) Keeping your torso still, pull both elbows upwards brushing the side of the body, and keep the forearms vertical. Squeeze your shoulder blades together at the end of the movement. Exhale as you pull.

4) Reverse the movement until your arms are straight, but keep the tension between your shoulder blades. Inhale as you lengthen the arms.

5) Aim for around 2 seconds up (concentric phase) and 2 seconds down (eccentric phase).

6) Repeat for the desired number of repetitions before safely placing the weights back onto the floor.

Key Points:

- Ensure you position your torso 30-40° from the floor to enable the desired muscles to pull the weights directly against gravity.
- Keep a neutral curve in your spine. Achieve this by tilting the pelvis fully forwards, then backwards, then finding a midpoint with a slight inward curve of your lower back (before you tip into position). Keep your core braced, chest open (& slightly lifted), and shoulders back and down.
- Breathe out as you pull, breathe in as you release.
- Keep your torso still and avoid becoming more upright as you pull.
- Consciously bring your shoulder blades together (and down) at the end of the pull.
- Your forearms should stay vertical throughout.

Single-Arm Row

Target Muscles: Latissimus Dorsi, Posterior Deltoid, Mid & Lower Trapezius, Rhomboids, Biceps

Outline: The Single-Arm Row is a great alternative if the Bent-Over Row puts excess stress or discomfort in the lower back. A bench is used to support the body's position. As with the other horizontal pulls, it strengthens the muscles of the back and biceps.

It is also another unilateral exercise, enabling you to focus on the quality of the movement on each side individually, without your stronger side being dominant. It also adds a core element to prevent unwanted rotation of the trunk.

As always, choose a lightweight to start with and only progress the load when you can comfortably perform 15+ repetitions with excellent technique.

Equipment: Bench and a Dumbbell or Kettlebell.

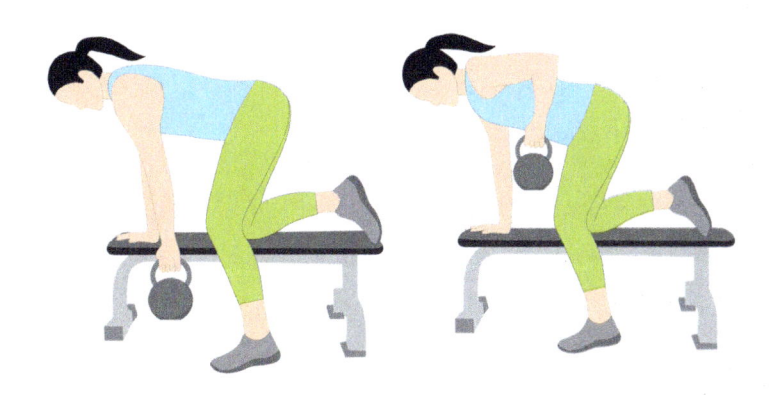

Single-Arm Row

Instructions:

1) Place your chosen weight to the right of the bench. Stand on the right side of the bench, behind the weight, and place your left knee on the bench, underneath your left hip. Move your right foot out to the side (in line with the opposite knee) until both sides of your pelvis are level.

2) Tip forward and place your left hand on the bench, approximately under the left shoulder. Unlock the elbow joint. Allow the right arm to hang under the right shoulder.

3) Brace the core and align the spine into its natural curves. Set the shoulder blades back and down, and tuck the chin so you are looking at the bench under your forehead. Reach for the weight with the right hand and then reset the shoulder blade back and down.

4) Keeping your torso still, pull the right elbow upwards brushing the side of the body, keeping the forearm vertical. Squeeze your shoulder blades together at the top of the movement. Exhale as you pull.

5) Reverse the movement until your arm is straight, but keep the tension between your shoulder blades. Inhale as you lengthen the arms.

6) Aim for around 2 seconds up (concentric phase) and 2 seconds down (eccentric phase).

7) Repeat for the desired number of repetitions before switching to the other side.

Key Points:

- Ensure you position your torso so the left/right sides of your pelvis are level and the shoulders are level.
- Keep a neutral curve in your spine. Achieve this by tilting the pelvis fully forwards, then backwards, then finding a midpoint with a slight inward curve of your lower back (before you start). Keep your core braced, chest open (& slightly lifted), and shoulders back and down.
- Breathe out as you pull, breathe in as you release.
- Keep your torso still and avoid twisting your trunk as you pull.
- Consciously bring your shoulder blade back (and down) at the end of the pull.
- Your forearm should stay vertical throughout.

Inverted Row

Target Muscles: Latissimus Dorsi, Posterior Deltoid, Mid & Lower Trapezius, Rhomboids, Biceps

Outline: The Inverted Row is a bodyweight exercise that can be adapted for all abilities, assuming the height of the required bar can be adjusted. You can also perform it using a suspension trainer such as a TRX®.

As with the other horizontal pull exercises, it works the back and biceps and also requires some core and glute engagement to keep the body aligned.

You perform it by positioning yourself under a fixed bar, face-up, and pulling your body weight up towards the bar. It is easiest when the bar is high and you are more upright, and hardest when the bar is low and you are closer to being horizontal. You can also adjust the difficulty by whether you keep your legs straight (more challenging), or bend at the knees (less challenging).

Start with a relatively easy option and progress when you can comfortably perform 15+ repetitions with great technique.

Equipment: Fixed bar such as a smith machine in a gym, *Lebert EQualizer* Bars, or a suspension trainer.

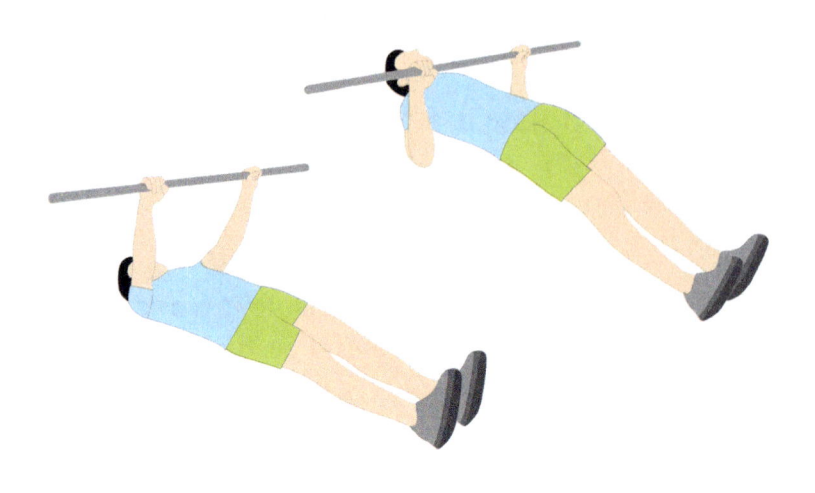

Inverted Row

Instructions:

1) Adjust your bar to the appropriate height. Grip the bar with either an overhand or underhand grip, shoulder-width apart. Lean back so your arms are straight, keeping the shoulder blades back and down. Lift your hips by engaging your glutes to achieve a straight line from your shoulders, through your hips, to your knees. Brace your core and keep your spine in its neutral curves.

2) Pull your elbows back, brushing the side of the body, lifting your torso towards the bar. The bar should meet your body just under your chest, around the lower ribs. If not, move your feet away, or towards the bar to correct it.

3) At the top of the movement, your forearms should be perpendicular (90°) to your body and the shoulder blades should be pulled back towards each other, and down the back. Exhale as you rise. Ensure the whole body stays in alignment throughout.

4) Lower yourself by extending the arms, keeping the glutes engaged to avoid the hips dropping towards the floor. Inhale as you lower yourself. At the bottom, keep tension in between the shoulder blades.

5) Aim for around 2 seconds up (concentric phase) and 2 seconds down (eccentric phase).

7) Repeat for the desired number of repetitions.

Key Points:

- Ensure you engage both your core and glutes throughout to align your body and keep a neutral spinal alignment.
- Keep a neutral curve in your spine. Achieve this by tilting the pelvis fully forwards, then backwards, then finding a midpoint with a slight inward curve of your lower back (before you start). Keep your core braced, chest open (& slightly lifted), and shoulders back and down.
- Breathe out as you pull, breathe in as you release.
- Consciously bring your shoulder blade back (and down) at the end of the pull.
- Your forearm should stay perpendicular to the body throughout.
- If using a suspension trainer such as the TRX®, use a neutral grip with the palms of the hands facing in towards each other.

Vertical Pull

A vertical row involves pulling handles/a bar towards you from above your head, or pulling your body towards an object (e.g. a bar) above your head.

Examples of vertical pulls include Close-Grip Pulldown, Lat Pulldown, Chin Ups, and Pull Ups.

Close-Grip Pulldown (Resistance Bands)

Target Muscles: Latissimus Dorsi, Posterior Deltoid, Mid & Lower Trapezius, Rhomboids, Biceps

Outline: This is a great starting point to increase strength in the back and bicep muscles through a vertical pull. Just as the Seated Band Row in the horizontal pull section; it is safe, simple and effective.

The fundamental difference between the two is that the Close-Grip Pulldown has a high anchor point, which results in your Latissimus Dorsi (Lats) being put into a lengthened position, allowing them to work through a greater range of motion (ROM). It also encourages more work from your Lower Trapezius, which creates scapula depression (the shoulder blades moving in a downward direction).

Minimal and affordable equipment is required, meaning you can do it at home or the gym, although it requires an anchor point that is relatively high (at least at the height of your outstretched arms above your head whilst standing).

Resistance bands come in various levels of resistance, allowing room to start easy and progress when required. Another way of progressing with resistance bands is to increase the stretch on the band before starting the exercise, by anchoring the band to a higher point...

Aim to progress the resistance, or the exercise, when you can perform 15+ repetitions with good technique.

Equipment: Chair or bench, 2 x resistance bands, and something sturdy to provide an anchor for the band.

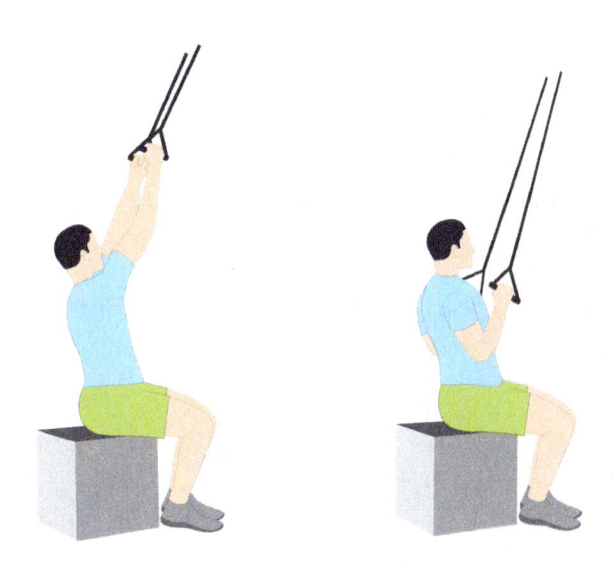

Close-Grip Pulldown (Resistance Bands)

Instructions:

1) Attach two resistance bands to a sturdy object as an anchor point, around the height of your fingertips when your arms are outstretched above your head, whilst standing. Sit on a chair or bench, facing the anchor point. Hold a band in each hand and ensure there is a slight stretch in the bands when the arms are outstretched. Set your feet shoulder-width with the ankles under the knees. Lean back slightly, roll the shoulders back and down, tuck the chin to keep the neck in its natural alignment and brace the core, creating a neutral spine.

2) Keeping your torso still, pull both elbows down brushing the side of the body, and keep the forearms pointing in the same direction as the bands. Squeeze your shoulder blades together, and down into your 'back pockets', at the end of the movement. Exhale as you pull.

3) Reverse the movement until your arms are straight, but keep the tension between your shoulder blades. Inhale as you lengthen the arms.

4) Aim for around 2 seconds down (concentric phase) and 2 seconds up (eccentric phase).

5) Repeat for the desired number of repetitions before leaning forward to create slack in the band before you let go!

Key Points:

- Ensure there is some tension in the bands throughout the full ROM. You don't want them to go slack at any point.
- Keep a neutral curve in your spine. Achieve this by tilting the pelvis fully forwards, then backwards, then finding a midpoint with a slight inward curve of your lower back (before you start). Keep your core braced, chest open (& slightly lifted), and shoulders relaxed back and down.
- Breathe out as you pull, breathe in as you release.
- Keep your torso still and avoid leaning back excessively or arching your back during the pull.
- Consciously bring your shoulder blades together and down at the end of the pull.
- Your forearms should stay in line with the bands throughout.
- You can also perform this exercise using a lat pulldown machine in the gym with a close-grip handle attachment.

Lat Pulldown (Machine)

Target Muscles: Latissimus Dorsi, Mid & Lower Trapezius, Rhomboids, Biceps

Outline: This exercise is very similar to the close-grip pulldown, but is performed with a wide grip. It is traditionally performed using a machine, but could also be performed using two resistance bands by anchoring them high, approximately one metre apart.

The wide grip changes the movement pattern slightly, causing more work in the Lats and less work in the Posterior Deltoid.

Using resistance bands makes it minimal and affordable in terms of equipment, making it more suitable for non-gym environments, but if using a gym, it is best performed using the machine.

You can adjust resistance in relatively small increments on the Lat Pulldown machine and should be progressed when you can perform 15+ repetitions with excellent technique.

Equipment: Lat Pulldown Machine or; chair/bench, two resistance bands, and a suitable anchor point.

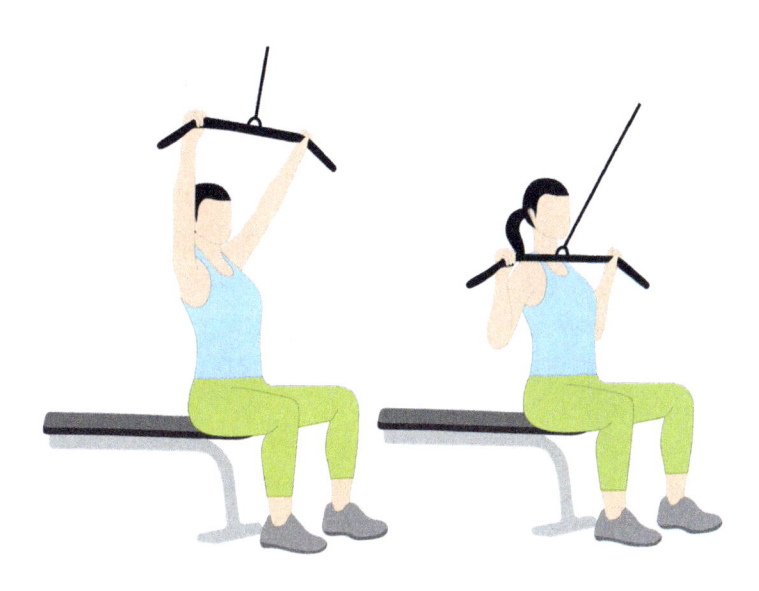

Lat Pulldown

Instructions (Lat Pulldown Machine):

1) Select an appropriate weight. Adjust the seat/thigh support so your ankles can be positioned under your knees, and the thighs are supported. Stand and grip the bar approximately 1.5 x shoulder width and return to the seated position. Lean back slightly, roll the

shoulders back and down, tuck the chin to keep the neck in its natural alignment and brace the core, creating a neutral spine.

2) Keeping your torso still, pull both elbows down to the side of the body, keeping the forearms close to vertical. Squeeze your shoulder blades together, and down into your 'back pockets', at the end of the movement. Exhale as you pull.

3) Reverse the movement until your arms are straight, but keep the tension between your shoulder blades. Inhale as you lengthen the arms.

4) Aim for around 2 seconds down (concentric phase) and 2 seconds up (eccentric phase).

5) Repeat for the desired number of repetitions before standing and resting the weights back onto the stack.

Key Points:

- Keep a neutral curve in your spine. Achieve this by tilting the pelvis fully forwards, then backwards, then finding a midpoint with a slight inward curve of your lower back (before you start). Keep your core braced, chest open (& slightly lifted), and shoulders relaxed back and down.
- Breathe out as you pull, breathe in as you release.
- Keep your torso still and avoid leaning back excessively or arching your back during the pull.
- Consciously bring your shoulder blades together and down at the end of the pull.
- Your forearms should stay close to vertical.
- You can also perform this exercise using two resistance bands with the same technique, but without a thigh support.

Chin Ups (Band Assisted)

Target Muscles: Latissimus Dorsi, Posterior Deltoid, Mid & Lower Trapezius, Rhomboids, Biceps

Outline: This exercise is very similar to the Close-Grip Pulldown in terms of movement pattern and muscles being used, but is more challenging to perform.

Minimal and affordable equipment is required, meaning you can do it at home or the gym, although it requires a pull up bar or fixed horizontal bar that can easily take your body weight.

Resistance bands come in various levels of resistance, allowing room to start easy (using a band with greater resistance to assist you) and progress when required to less assistance through bands with less resistance.

Aim to lower the assistance level through a lighter resistance band once you can perform 15+ repetitions with good technique.

Equipment: Pull Up Bar or fixed horizontal bar, and a resistance band.

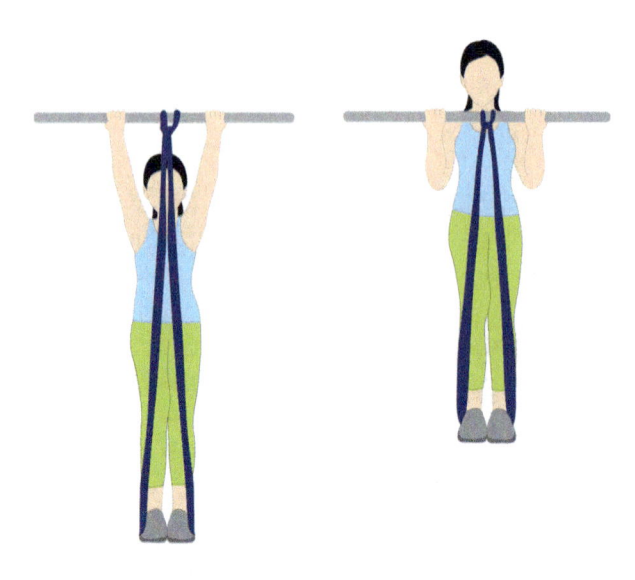

Band-Assisted Chin Ups

Instructions:

1) Attach the resistance band to the middle of the bar by placing the band over the bar, passing one end through the loop at the other end, and pulling tight. Step one foot into the band, place both hands on the bar shoulder-width apart, with your palms facing towards you (underhand grip). Place the second foot into the band. Set the shoulder blades back and down, look straight ahead and brace the core.

2) Keeping your core braced and spine neutral, pull both elbows down brushing the side of the body, and keep the forearms vertical until your chin is above the bar. Squeeze your shoulder blades together, and down into your 'back pockets', at the end of the movement. Exhale as you pull.

3) Reverse the movement until your arms are straight, but keep the tension between your shoulder blades. Inhale as you lengthen the arms.

4) Aim for around 1-2 seconds up (concentric phase) and 2 seconds down (eccentric phase).

5) Repeat for the desired number of repetitions before stepping out of the band one foot at a time.

Key Points:

- Ensure you are using bands that are specifically for Assisted Pull Ups because of their additional durability.
- Keep a neutral curve in your spine. Achieve this by tilting the pelvis fully forwards, then backwards, then finding a midpoint with a slight inward curve of your lower back (before you start). Keep your core braced, chest open (& slightly lifted), and shoulders relaxed back and down.
- Breathe out as you pull up, breathe in as you release.
- Keep your torso still and avoid leaning back excessively or arching your back during the pull.
- Consciously bring your shoulder blades together and down at the end of the pull.
- Your forearms should stay vertical throughout.
- You can also perform this exercise unassisted if capable or using an Assisted Chin/Pull Up Machine in a gym.

Pull Ups (Band Assisted)

Target Muscles: Latissimus Dorsi, Mid & Lower Trapezius, Rhomboids, Biceps

Outline: This exercise is very similar to the Assisted Chin Ups, but is performed with a wide, overhand grip. The wide, overhand grip changes the movement pattern slightly, causing more work in the Lats and less work in the Posterior Deltoid.

The equipment requirements and the progression/regressions are the same as the Assisted Chin Ups above.

Aim to lower the assistance level through a lighter resistance band once you can perform 15+ repetitions with good technique.

Equipment: Pull up bar or fixed horizontal bar, and a resistance band.

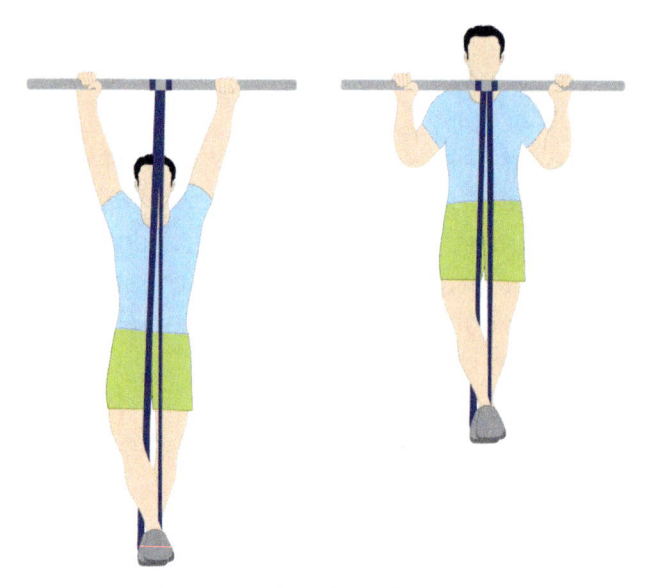

Band-Assisted Pull Ups

Instructions:

1) Attach the resistance band to the middle of the bar by placing the band over the bar, passing one end through the loop at the other end, and pulling tight. Step one foot into the band, and place both hands on the bar with an overhand grip (palms away from you), approximately 1.5 x shoulder width. Place the second foot into the band. Set the shoulder blades back and down, look straight ahead and brace the core.

2) Keeping your core braced and spine neutral, pull both elbows down into the side of the body, keeping the forearms close to vertical. Squeeze your shoulder blades together, and down into your 'back pockets' at the end of the movement. Exhale as you pull.

3) Reverse the movement until your arms are straight, but keep the tension between your shoulder blades. Inhale as you lengthen the arms.

4) Aim for around 1-2 seconds up (concentric phase) and 2 seconds down (eccentric phase).

5) Repeat for the desired number of repetitions before stepping out of the band one foot at a time.

Key Points:

- Ensure you are using bands that are specifically for assisted pull ups due to their additional durability.
- Keep a neutral curve in your spine. Achieve this by tilting the pelvis fully forwards, then backwards, then finding a midpoint with a slight inward curve of your lower back (before you start). Keep your core braced, chest open (& slightly lifted), and shoulders relaxed back and down.
- Breathe out as you pull up, breathe in as you release.
- Keep your torso still and avoid leaning back excessively or arching your back during the pull.
- Consciously bring your shoulder blades together and down at the end of the pull.
- Your forearms should stay close to vertical throughout.
- This exercise can also be performed unassisted if capable or using an Assisted Chin/Pull Up Machine in a gym.

The 'Push'

An exercise must meet all the following criteria to be categorized as a 'push':

- Upper body movement
- Compound (2 or more moving joints)
- Involve pressing or pushing a load away from the upper body, or the upper body moving away from a fixed surface during the push/press

Push exercises predominantly utilize the muscles of the chest (Pec Major), shoulders (Deltoids) and the back of the arms (Triceps). It is an important movement pattern in everyday life as it enables us to perform functional tasks such as pushing ourselves up off the floor (before we can use our legs to stand), opening self-closing (swing) doors, and lifting objects onto tall shelves.

Despite its important role in daily movement patterns, it's advisable to avoid the overuse of push exercises because the chest (pectorals) and the front of the shoulder (anterior deltoids) are commonly overactive/tight muscles, leading to poor posture. Over-training these muscles, compared to their opposing muscles, can exacerbate postural problems and lead to injury.

I have separated the push into two separate exercise categories: *the horizontal push* and *the vertical push*. This helps to provide a more balanced training outcome because of the difference in primary muscles used between the horizontal and vertical push, and muscles working through varied 'planes of motion' (direction of movement), as well as preventing overuse of potentially short/overactive muscles.

The Horizontal Push

A horizontal push involves pushing a weight out in front of your body, or pushing your body away from a surface or object in front of your chest. These movement patterns predominantly work the pectorals, front deltoids, and triceps.

Examples of a horizontal push include; Push Ups (or Press Ups!), Chest Press (Machine/Cables/Resistance Bands/TRX), Barbell Bench Press, and Dumbbell Bench Press.

Push Up (Press Up)

Target Muscles: Pectoralis Major, Anterior Deltoid, Triceps, Core

Outline: The Push Up, or Press Up, is a great bodyweight exercise for the chest and the back of the arms, and can be performed almost anywhere.

There are various levels of difficulty making it suitable for most people. It's important to find the version that is most suitable for you, and then work through the progressions.

As a guide, I would suggest focusing on the version in which you can perform a minimum of 8 repetitions, but not over 15. If you can't manage 8, regress to an easier version. If you can do over 15 (with excellent technique), progress to a harder version.

Equipment: None, Mat, Raised Bench, Wall (dependant upon the version being performed).

The images show progressive versions from easiest to hardest.

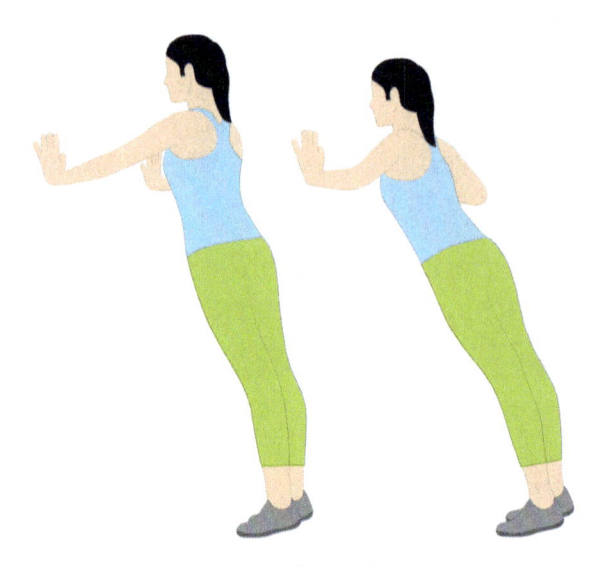

Wall Push Ups

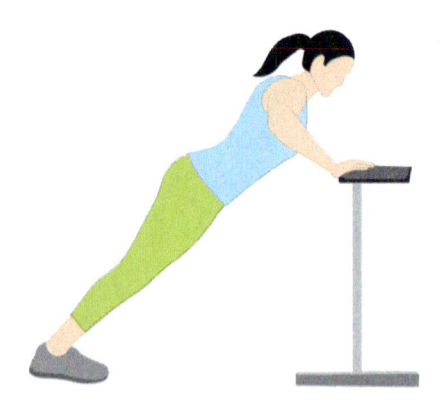

Raised Push Ups

THE ESSENTIAL EIGHT 123

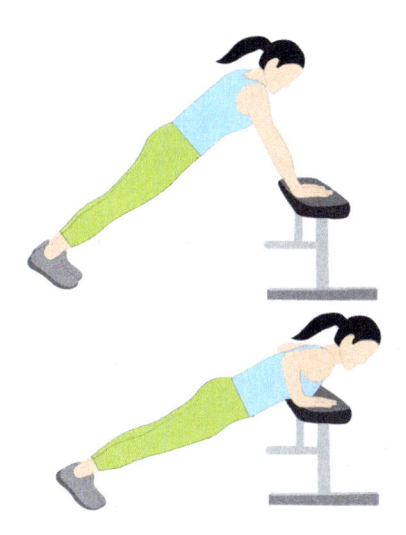

Raised Push Ups (Lower)

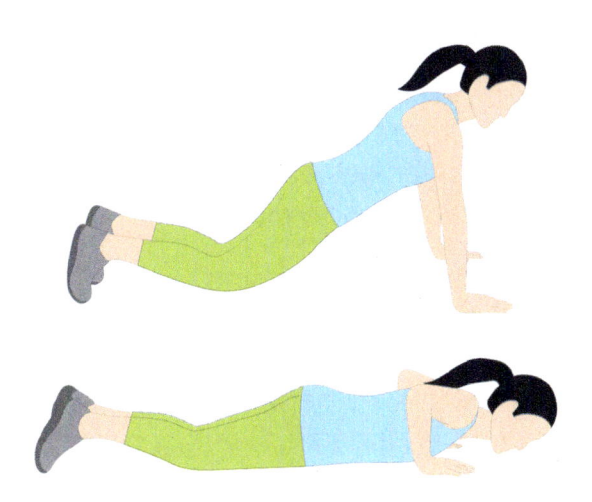

¾ Push Ups

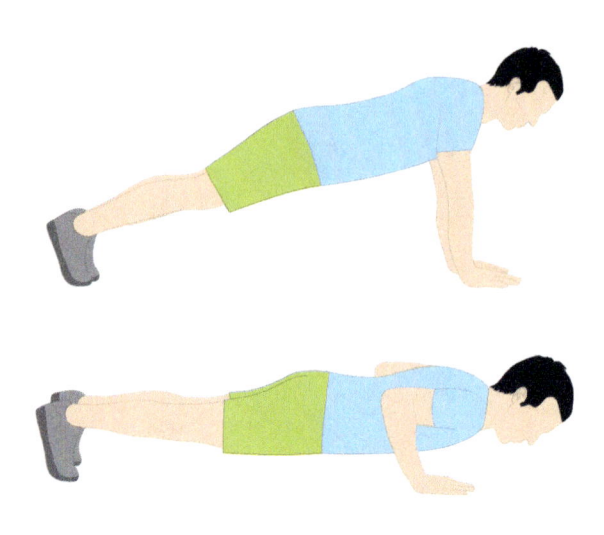

Full Push Ups

Instructions:

1) Either place your knees, or feet, on the floor and place your hands on the surface being used. Your hands should be just outside shoulder width and in line with your lower chest. Unlock the elbows, engage your glutes and brace your core, creating a straight line through your body from ankles or knees, through the hips, to the shoulders. Keep your neck in line with the rest of the spine.

2) Keeping your core braced and spine neutral, lower your body until your upper arms are parallel to the floor, or a little lower if possible. At the bottom of the Push Up, the elbows should be over the wrists so your forearms are perpendicular (at 90° to) your torso, and parallel to each other. Inhale as you descend.

3) Press your palms into the surface you are using, pushing your torso away from the chosen surface and extending the arms until you have a very slight bend left in them. Keep tension between your shoulder blades to maintain the stability of the shoulder girdle

(shoulder blades and collarbones). Exhale as you lengthen the arms.

4) Aim for around 2 seconds up (concentric phase) and 2 seconds down (eccentric phase).

5) Repeat for the desired number of repetitions before resting.

Key Points:

- Hand positioning is key... check at the bottom of the Push Up, that your forearms are perpendicular to the body, parallel to each other, and in line with your mid-lower chest. If someone photographed your back during the Push Up, your torso and upper arms should create an arrow shape (see image below).

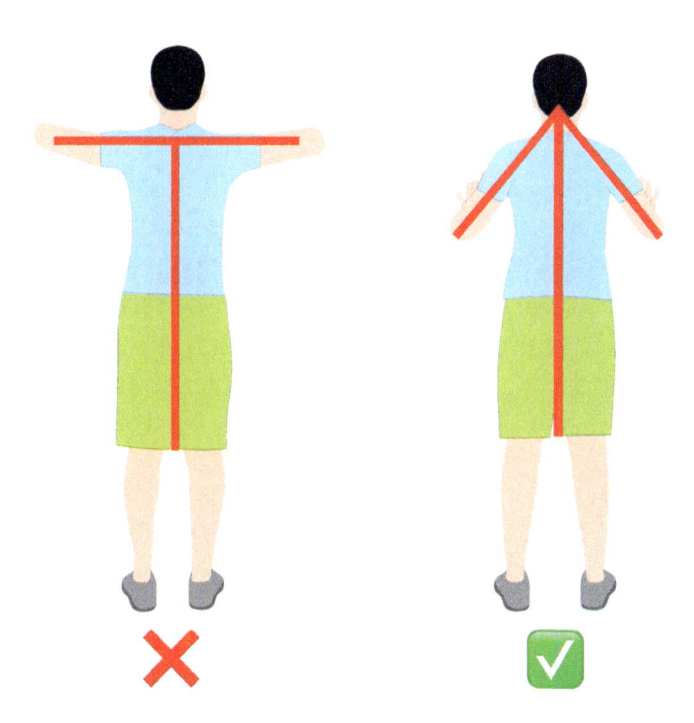

Arm Position During Push Ups

- Keep a neutral curve in your spine. Achieve this by tilting the pelvis fully forwards, then backwards, then finding a midpoint with a slight inward curve of your lower back (before you start). Keep your core braced, chest open (& slightly lifted), and shoulder blades back and down.
- Breathe out as you push up, breathe in as you lower.
- Keep your body aligned; avoid your hips rising or descending out of alignment between knees and shoulders.
- Create stability at the shoulder by keeping tension between the shoulder blades, and feeling a subtle external screwing of your hands on the floor/bench/wall (without them physically moving).

Dumbbell Bench Press

Target Muscles: Pectoralis Major, Anterior Deltoid, Triceps

Outline: This exercise utilizes the same muscles as the Push Up, but uses dumbbells instead of bodyweight. This has its advantages and disadvantages; the disadvantages include the necessity of dumbbells and a bench, requiring either the purchase of them for home use, or gym access, and the decreased demand on the core muscles compared to the Push Up. The advantages include; increased stability demands at the shoulder, and simpler methods of regression and progression (simply decreasing or increasing the weight of the dumbbells) compared to the Push Ups.

If you can do over 15 repetitions (with good technique), you will need to progress the weight of the dumbbells. If you would rather focus on increased core demand, shoulder stability, and left-right muscle balance rather than increased weight, you can progress by performing the exercise with alternating arms, and then the Single-Arm Dumbbell Bench Press.

No access to a bench? It is possible to do a floor press, where you simply perform the same exercise lying on a mat.

Equipment: Dumbbells and a bench.

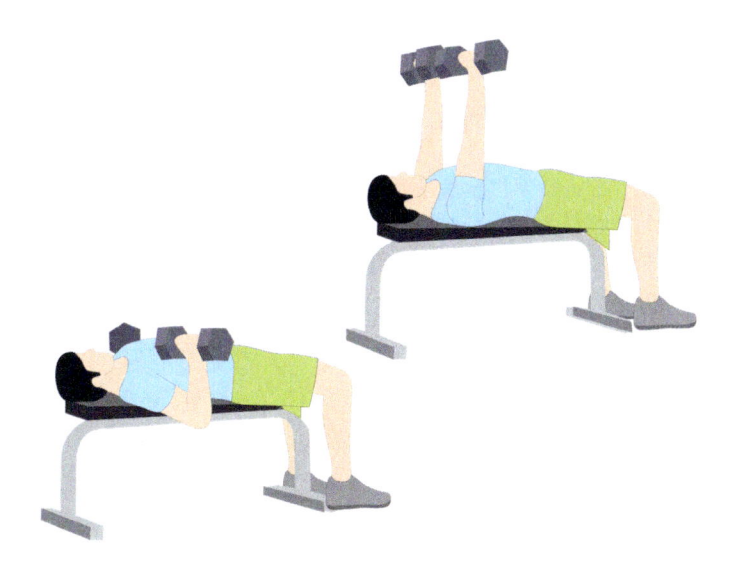

Dumbbell Bench Press

Instructions:

1) Pick up a dumbbell in each hand (safely, without arching your back) and lie down on a bench, placing the dumbbells close to your armpits with the elbows under the wrists. Place the feet shoulder-width with ankles under knees. Brace your core and press the dumbbells over the chest until the arms are straight (elbows slightly bent), your palms are pointing toward your feet, your wrists are in neutral alignment, and your shoulder blades are back and down.

2) Keeping your core braced and spine neutral, lower the dumbbells, allowing them to separate so the wrists stay over the elbows. The dumbbells should remain in line with the mid-chest, the elbows finish level with the bench, and your upper arms are approximately 45° angle from your body. Inhale as the dumbbells descend.

3) Press the dumbbells back to the top position, keeping a slight gap between them at the top. Maintain some tension between your shoulder blades to stabilise the shoulder girdle and exhale as the dumbbells rise.

4) Aim for around 2 seconds up (concentric phase) and 2 seconds down (eccentric phase).

5) Repeat for the desired number of repetitions before returning the dumbbells towards the armpits, carefully sitting back up, and placing the dumbbells safely back down.

Key Points:

- Keep a neutral curve in your spine. Achieve this by tilting the pelvis fully forwards, then backwards, then finding a midpoint with a slight inward curve of your lower back (before you start). Keep your core braced, chest open (& slightly lifted), and shoulder blades back and down.
- Breathe out as you push the dumbbells up. Breathe in as you lower them.
- Ensure your wrists always stay over the elbows, and check you have approximately a 45° angle between the torso and upper arm at the bottom of the exercise.
- Create stability at the shoulder by keeping tension between the shoulder blades.
- Avoid locking out the elbows at the top and keep a gap between the dumbbells to keep tension in the muscles.
- From a side view, keep the dumbbells aligned with the chest.

The Vertical Push

A vertical push involves pushing weight overhead. This predominantly works the deltoids and triceps.

Examples of a vertical push are variations of a Shoulder Press or Overhead Press and include; Shoulder Press (Machine/Cables/Resistance Bands), Barbell Overhead Press, Dumbbell Shoulder (or 'Military') Press, and Kettlebell Overhead Press.

Dumbbell Shoulder Press

Target Muscles: Deltoids and Triceps

Outline: The Dumbbells Shoulder Press, sometimes referred to as a Military Press, predominantly works the shoulders and the back of the arms by pressing dumbbells vertically overhead.

When using relatively heavy dumbbells, it can be a little tricky to transition them into the start position. View the Exercise Video Library (Bonus Material) to see how to perform a "Dumbbell Clean" to get them into the start position.

You can choose to perform this exercise seated or standing. If you experience any adverse shoulder discomfort whilst performing the Dumbbell Shoulder Press, I suggest attempting the Kettlebell Overhead Press outlined next.

As always, if you can complete over 15 repetitions (with good technique), you will need to progress the weight of the dumbbells.

Equipment: Dumbbells (and a bench or chair for the seated version).

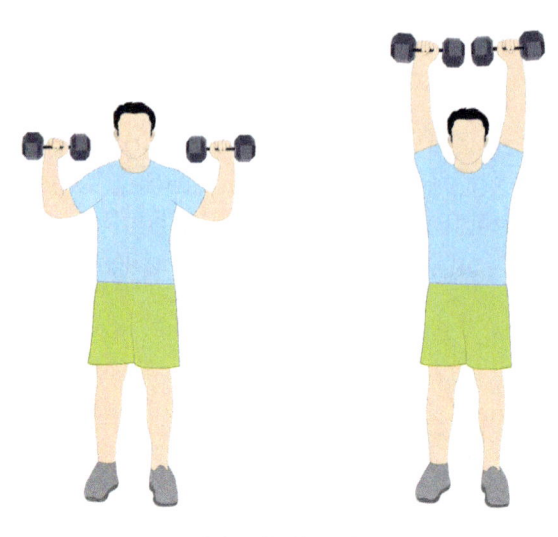

Dumbbell Shoulder Press

Instructions:

1) Pick up a dumbbell in each hand (safely, without arching your back) and position them just in front of your shoulders with your elbows under your wrists. Either sit or stay standing. Place the feet hip-shoulder width apart. Look straight ahead, brace your core and press the dumbbells overhead until the arms are straight (elbows slightly bent) and in line with your ears, your palms are pointing forward, your wrists are in neutral alignment, and your shoulder blades are back and down.

2) Keeping your core braced and spine neutral, lower the dumbbells, allowing them to separate so the wrists stay over the elbows until the dumbbells reach the height of your jaw. From a side view, a line between the two dumbbells would pass through your cheeks. Inhale as the dumbbells descend.

3) Press the dumbbells back overhead, keeping a slight gap between them at the top, and exhale as the dumbbells rise. Stack

the joints (shoulder/elbow/wrist) on top of each other from a side view, in line with the ears (or just in front if necessary).

4) Aim for around 2 seconds up (concentric phase) and 2 seconds down (eccentric phase).

5) Repeat for the desired number of repetitions before returning the dumbbells towards the front of the shoulders, flipping your elbows over the top of the dumbbells and lowering them back down before placing them safely onto the floor.

Key Points:

- Keep a neutral curve in your spine. Achieve this by tilting the pelvis fully forwards, then backwards, then finding a midpoint with a slight inward curve of your lower back (before you start). Keep your core braced, chest open (& slightly lifted), and shoulder blades back and down.
- Breathe out as you press the dumbbells up. Breathe in as you lower them.
- Ensure your wrists always stay over the elbows throughout the exercise.
- Avoid locking out the elbows at the top and keep a gap between the dumbbells to keep tension in the muscles. Lower them to around jaw height for a full range of motion.
- From a side view, keep the dumbbells aligned with the ears/back of the jaw.

Kettlebell Overhead Press

Target Muscles: Deltoids and Triceps

Outline: The Kettlebell Overhead Press is another great exercise for the shoulders and the back of the arms. It can be performed 1 arm at a time (unilaterally) or both arms at the same time (bilaterally). We are going to focus on the unilateral version because it only requires one kettlebell, makes it easier to get the kettlebell into the start position, is a little more functional, and we have already looked at a bilateral overhead press above.

When using a relatively heavy kettlebell, it can be a little tricky to get it into the start position. View the Exercise Video Library (Bonus Material) to see how to perform a "Kettlebell Clean" to get it into the start position. This start position is known as 'the rack' in kettlebell training.

As always, if you can complete over 15 repetitions (with good technique), you will need to progress the weight of the dumbbells.

Equipment: Kettlebell.

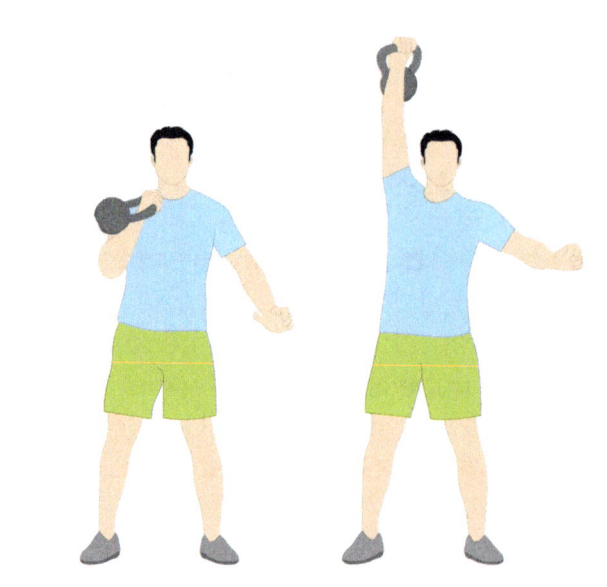

Single-Arm Kettlebell Overhead Press

Instructions:

1) Pick up a kettlebell in one hand (safely, without arching your back) and position it in the rack position; elbow into the ribs, palm towards the sternum (breastbone) facing across your body, forearm angled in towards the middle of the chest. You can use

your other hand to help you maneuver the kettlebell into the rack position, or watch the instruction video on how to do it through the kettlebell clean.

2) Set your feet hip-shoulder width, unlock your knees, brace your core, and set the shoulder blades back and down. Look straight ahead and take a breath in.

3) As you exhale, press the kettlebell straight up overhead, turning your palms forward. Keep a slight bend in the elbow at the top with the shoulder/elbow/wrists stacked on top of each other from a side view.

4) Lower the kettlebell back to the rack position via a vertical path (straight line down), finishing back with the palm facing across the body, close to the sternum, with the elbow into the ribs. Inhale as you descend.

5) Aim for around 1-2 seconds up (concentric phase) and 2 seconds down (eccentric phase).

6) Repeat for the desired number of repetitions before switching to the other side.

Key Points:

- Keep a neutral curve in your spine. Achieve this by tilting the pelvis fully forwards, then backwards, then finding a midpoint with a slight inward curve of your lower back (before you start). Keep your core braced, chest open (& slightly lifted), and shoulder blades back and down.
- Breathe out as you press the kettlebell up and breathe in as you lower it.
- Move the kettlebell through a vertical path, straight line up and straight line down.
- Avoid locking out the elbows at the top, and finish with the palm facing forward.
- From a side view, stack the joints (shoulder/elbow/wrist) on top of each other when the kettlebell is overhead.

- You can keep your grip closed, or open, whichever is preferred.

ADDITIONAL PUSH: DIPS

Dips are a bit of an anomaly and don't fit perfectly in either the *'horizontal push'* or *'vertical push'* categories. The 'push' occurs in more of a downward direction, so it would make sense to put it into the *'vertical push'* category, but the muscles worked are more like those working in the *'horizontal push'*!

I wanted to include it as another push because of the minimal equipment required, the functionality of pushing yourself up from low sitting positions (for those of you preparing a strong, healthy body for your later years), and the ability to perform it almost anywhere.

It focuses a lot of work on the back of the arms, but also utilizes the muscles at the front of the shoulder and the chest.

Bodyweight Bench Dips

Target Muscles: Triceps, Anterior Deltoid, Pectoralis Major

Outline: You can perform Bodyweight Bench Dips using a bench, sofa, sturdy chair, bed, fixed bar, or anything else that is secure at the right height.

If you find them too challenging, you can simply bend your knees more, bringing your feet closer to the bench, or if you find them too easy, you can simply straighten the legs out, or progress onto full bodyweight dips on parallel bars.

As a guide, I would suggest focusing on a body position that enables you to perform a minimum of 8 repetitions, but not over 15. If you can't manage 8, regress to an easier body position. If you can do over 15 (with great technique), progress to a harder body position.

Equipment: Bench, or similar.

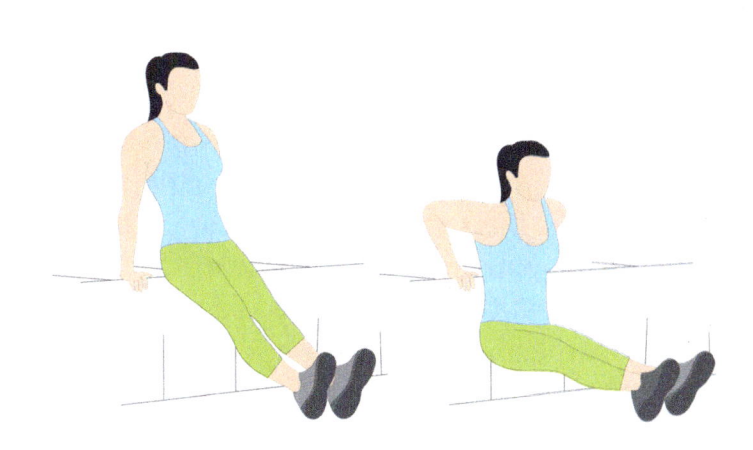

Bodyweight Dips

Instructions:

1) Sit on the edge of a bench with your hands placed by your sides, palms on the bench (close to the front edge), with your thumbs pointing forwards and fingers angled away from your sides. Lift your chest, set your shoulder blades back and down, and look straight ahead. Place your feet hip-width apart at your chosen distance from the bench (closer = easier, further = harder). Push your hands into the bench, lift your bum off the bench and hover it over the edge.

2) Lower your bum towards the floor by bending your elbows and moving them behind your shoulders until your upper arms are horizontal. Inhale as your body lowers. Keep your chest open and shoulders down.

3) Press your palms on the bench, straightening your arms and raising your body away from the floor. Straighten your arms without hyper-extending your elbows at the top. Exhale as you rise.

4) Aim for around 2 seconds up (concentric phase) and 2 seconds down (eccentric phase).

5) Repeat for the desired number of repetitions before resting your bum back on the bench.

Key Points:

- Angle your fingers away from the sides of your body to put the shoulder joint into a more desirable position, with your chest open and shoulder blades back and down.
- Breathe out as you push up, breathe in as you lower.
- Create stability at the shoulder by keeping tension between the shoulder blades, and feeling a subtle external screwing of your hands on the bench (without them physically moving).

The Carry

To be categorized as a "carry", an exercise must involve walking (potentially jogging/running) whilst holding a weight with the upper body. We would consider them to be a total body strength training exercise, as multiple muscles within both the upper and lower body are under load.

As well as being great for improving overall strength (and endurance), carries are superb for improving grip strength and our ability to perform activities of daily living in our later years, such as carrying shopping or carrying children/grandchildren. It's all very well being able to lift, push and pull loads, but our daily activities often involve walking with those loads as well.

Carries are also great for core strength when performed unilaterally with the load held on one side of the body.

Farmer's Walk

Target Muscles: Total body, including grip strength

Outline: The Farmer's Walk is a great starting point for carries. It is an excellent total body strength and endurance activity that also improves grip strength and can also have a positive impact on the cardiovascular system.

You can perform it with dumbbells, kettlebells, or any weight that can be held by the sides of the body. You will need one for each hand of equal weight.

Rather than repetitions, you can monitor it through distance walked, number of steps, or time. If you choose to carry lighter weights and focus on more distance/time, your results will be more muscular endurance based. Whereas, if you decide to carry heavier weights and focus on a shorter distance/time, your results will be more muscular strength-based.

I recommend using weights that challenge you for 30s of walking, progressing time with the same weight until you can complete 1 minute of walking, then progressing to heavier weights and repeating the process.

Equipment: Dumbbells or Kettlebells.

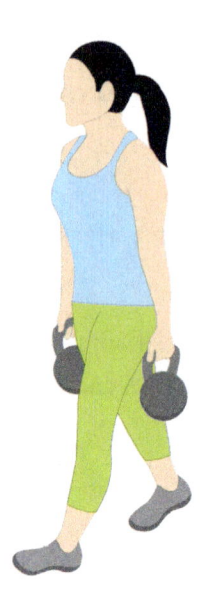

Farmer's Walk

Instructions:

1) Deadlift the dumbbells or kettlebells off the floor.

2) Grip the weights by the sides of your body, set your shoulders back and down, look straight ahead and brace your core. Walk in straight lines, back and fore if you need to, keeping your torso as upright as possible.

3) Once the time or distance is up, or when you can no longer hold the weights, safely place them down without rounding/bending the spine.

Key Points:

- Wrap the thumb around the handles for a full grip. Maintain an open chest with shoulder blades back and down.
- Keep a neutral curve in your spine. Achieve this by tilting the pelvis fully forwards, then backwards, then finding a midpoint

with a slight inward curve of your lower back (before you tip into position). Keep your core braced to maintain the alignment.
- Breathe naturally.
- Keep your torso steady, avoiding excessive rocking or swinging.
- Your arms should stay vertical next to your body throughout.

Suitcase Walk

Target Muscles: Total body, including grip and core strength

Outline: The Suitcase Walk is very similar to the Farmer's Walk, but you hold the weight in one hand only. This has the additional advantage of engaging your core muscles to prevent lateral flexion (side bending) of the spine. It also means that you can still perform it if you don't have access to two of the same weights.

You can perform it with dumbbells, kettlebells, or any weight that can be held by the side of the body.

As with the Farmer's Walk, you can monitor it through distance, the number of steps, or time. If you choose to carry lighter weights and focus on more distance/time, your results will be more muscular endurance based. Whereas, if you decide to carry heavier weights and focus on a shorter distance/time, your results will be more muscular strength-based.

I recommend using a weight that challenges you for 20-30s of walking per side, progressing time with the same weight until you can complete 1 minute per side, then progressing to heavier weights and repeating the process.

Equipment: Dumbbell or Kettlebell.

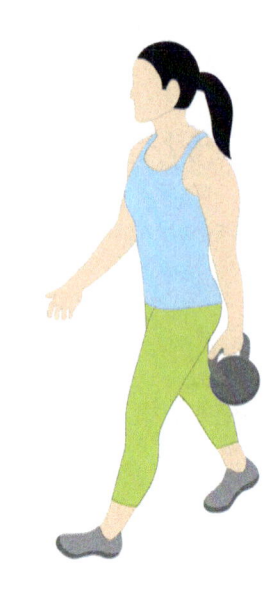

Suitcase Walk

Instructions:

1) Perform a Suitcase Deadlift to lift the dumbbell or kettlebell off the floor.

2) Grip the weight by the side of your body, set your shoulders back and down, look straight ahead and brace your core. Walk in straight lines, back and fore if you need to, keeping your torso as upright as possible.

3) Switch the weight to the other arm and repeat the same distance/time. Once the time or distance is up, or when you can no longer hold the weight, safely place it down without rounding/bending the spine.

Key Points:

- Wrap the thumb around the handle for a full grip. Maintain an open chest with shoulder blades back and down.

- Keep a neutral curve in your spine. Achieve this by tilting the pelvis fully forwards, then backwards, then finding a midpoint with a slight inward curve of your lower back (before you tip into position). Keep your core braced to maintain the alignment.
- Breathe naturally.
- Keep your torso steady, avoiding excessive rocking, swinging, or tilting to the side of the weight.
- Your arm should stay vertical next to your body throughout.
- Allow your spare arms to swing naturally.

Rack Walk

Target Muscles: Total body, including core strength.

Outline: The Rack Walk is another one-side carry, but you hold the weight in the 'rack' position as outlined in the Kettlebell Overhead Press. There is no grip strength in the Rack Walk, but eliminating this element stops it from being a limiting factor, allowing you to focus on the other benefits of the exercise. It enhances core strength but does not place the same demands on the core to prevent spinal lateral flexion, compared to the Suitcase Walk.

It is best performed using a kettlebell but can be replaced by a dumbbell if necessary.

As with the previous two carries, you can monitor it through distance walked, number of steps, or time. If you choose to carry lighter weights and focus on more distance/time, your results will be more muscular endurance based. Whereas, if you decide to carry heavier weights and focus on a shorter distance/time, your results will be more muscular strength-based.

I recommend using a weight that challenges you for 20-30s of walking per side, progressing time with the same weight until you can complete 1 minute per side, then progressing to heavier weights and repeating the process.

Equipment: Kettlebells (or Dumbbell).

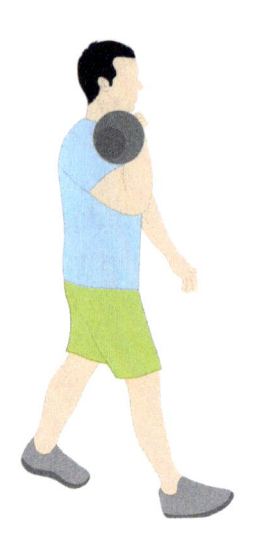

Rack Walk

Instructions:

1) Perform a Suitcase Deadlift to lift the kettlebell off the floor.

2) Transition the Kettlebell into the rack position, either through the help of the spare hand or through the Kettlebell Clean shown in the exercise video library.

2) Set your shoulders back and down, look straight ahead and brace your core. Walk in straight lines, back and fore if you need to, keeping your torso as upright as possible.

3) Switch the weight to the other arm and repeat the same distance/time. Once the time or distance is up, or when you can no longer hold the weight, safely place it down without rounding/bending the spine.

Key Points:

- Use either a closed grip or open palm. Maintain an open chest with shoulder blades back and down.

- Keep a neutral curve in your spine. Achieve this by tilting the pelvis fully forwards, then backwards, then finding a midpoint with a slight inward curve of your lower back (before you tip into position). Keep your core braced to maintain the alignment.
- Breathe naturally.
- Keep your torso steady, avoiding excessive rocking, swinging, or tilting to the side.
- Allow your spare arms to swing naturally.

The Essential Eight Summary

The Essential Eight should form the foundation of your weight training program.

There are more exercises that fit into the Essential Eight movements, but I have specifically chosen the exercises above as the most appropriate for those over 50. The aim is to go through a period of conditioning and mastering the general techniques before progressing on to alternatives or more advanced exercises.

For example, in the Squat section, I deliberately left out one of the most common squats; the *Barbell Back Squat*. This is mainly because of the spinal loading that occurs when you have a weight on the top of your back, as well as the potential need for a Squat Rack or technical skills needed to get the bar onto the back without a Squat Rack.

Performing a Squat that involves spinal loading is a potentially high-risk version to do if you have not yet mastered the technique involved in the Squat movement pattern. It is also relatively high risk for those of you in your 60s and beyond due to potential losses in bone density and changes in spinal curvature. So mastering the technique of the *Chair Squat, Bodyweight Squat, Goblet Squat,* and *Powerbag Front Squat* should be your priority before advancing onto Back Squats with a Powerbag or Barbell.

This is just one example within *The Essential Eight*, but there is a logical and scientific rationale behind all of my exercise choices within this book. However, to give you the best of both worlds, and ensure the options are there when you want them, I have included further alternatives and progressions in the exercise video library.

Chapter 12

8 Week Program

To support you in putting the content of this book into practice, I have produced an 8 week beginner program for you to follow. There is also a printable PDF version in the bonus material.

Before we get to the 8 week program, I want to recap on some of the terminology that I refer to in the programs, and also cover some key information on the planning and progression of your strength training.

Terminology Reminder

Repetitions (reps): how many times you perform an exercise. '10 reps' means that you perform the exercise 10 times before stopping and resting.

Sets: a set is a group of repetitions. 2 sets of 10 reps = 10 reps - rest - 10 reps - exercise finished.

Load: the 'weight' of the equipment that the muscles are producing force against. E.g. weight of a barbell or dumbbells.

Rest: the time taken to rest and recover between sets.

To provide yourself with the tools needed to progress appropriately to your individual needs, let's have a look at strength training planning and progression.

Planning

Frequency

The World Health Organization (WHO) recommends that adults (aged 18-64) and older adults (aged 65+) should perform muscle-strengthening activities at a moderate or greater intensity that involve all major muscle groups on 2 or more days a week.

Based on this, I recommend 2-3 sessions per week of strength training, combined with additional exercise that targets other components of fitness covered in the rest of the *Simple Fitness After 50* Series.

Volume

I'm a strong believer in quality over quantity when it comes to strength training.

The essential eight movement patterns outlined in this book give you a foundation for safe, effective, no-nonsense strength training exercises and should form the basis of your muscle-strengthening activities.

I recommend 20-60 minutes, including warm up and cool own activities per session. Volume is a variable that can be progressed, therefore I suggest starting with 20 minute sessions and increasing volume when you feel conditioned enough to do so.

Exercise Selection

Plan your exercises as per the example 8 week program, so that on a weekly basis you are creating a balance between the number of *pull* exercises versus the number of *push* exercises.

Include a variety of *hip hinge, squat,* and *step up* activities throughout each week, and include a '*carry*' in each session.

Exercises within each of *the essential eight* categories vary in difficulty. Start with the easier versions, those that are outlined at the beginning of each category in Chapter 11, and aim to increase the difficulty as and when you feel ready. There are additional exercises in the video exercise library which you can access through the bonus material.

Exercise Order

The 8 week programs are ordered in a logical sequence to give working muscles some recovery time before being used again.

They also mostly alternate between lower body and upper body exercises. This will provide your body with a cardiovascular benefit as the heart has to distribute blood to working muscles in different areas of the body each time you change exercise. This is referred to as Peripheral Heart Action (PHA).

Reps

As outlined earlier in the book, the number of repetitions and the associated load lifted in a strength training exercise changes the training effect.

Lifting very heavy for <6 reps improves your ability to lift very heavy objects very few times. This is termed Muscular Strength. Lifting low weights for >12 reps improves your ability to overcome light loads multiple times. This is termed Muscular Endurance.

In between these two, in the 6-12 rep range is hypertrophy training. This range focuses on increasing muscle mass, increasing resting metabolic rate and therefore fat loss through increased daily energy expenditure, as well as some gains in muscular strength and muscular endurance.

Avoiding very heavy loads and very high repetitions also minimizes the risk of injury associated with strength training.

Based on this, I recommend focusing on a broad range of 8-15 repetitions. With the higher end of 12-15 reps being less challenging due to the relatively lighter loads lifted, and the lower end of 8-10 reps seen as more challenging due to the relatively higher loads lifted.

Whenever you attempt a new exercise, perform it with no/low weight and at the higher end of the 8-15 rep range to learn the exercise through more repetition.

Sets

I have planned for 2 sets on your 8 week example programs, primarily to focus on quality over quantity, and time efficiency. Two good quality sets will be more effective than 3 mediocre sets. However, if you have time and feel you would benefit from performing a third set, then go ahead. Anything beyond 3 sets is unnecessary for most people.

It's important to think about the balance between push and pull exercises, though. If you change to 3 sets of the *push* exercise(s) then you need to change to 3 sets of the *pull* exercise(s) too.

Intensity

Once you've decided on the number of repetitions you'll perform, and you have mastered the technique of an exercise, it's important to apply the *principle of progressive overload* to your training, to ensure you maximise your results.

The *principle of progressive overload* simply states that unless you provide your body with a stimulus that is above and beyond what it's used to, it will not adapt.

In strength training, this means that it needs to be a challenge to complete the full set with good technique. If you get the intensity right, you should be able to complete the set but feel you cannot complete more repetitions.

If you finish the set and feel you could have continued, with good technique, then you should increase the load on the next set or session to increase the intensity. If you cannot finish the set without your technique deteriorating, lower the load slightly on the next set or session.

Rest

A standard rest period between sets, for a rep range of 8-15, is 1-2 minutes. I would suggest you base this on how hard you are working in the exercises, your fitness levels, and whether you are aiming to keep your heart rate up for cardiovascular benefits.

Reasons to keep the rest period around 1 minute include; you're lifting light weights to focus on technique, you have relatively high fitness levels, and/or you're aiming to keep your heart rate elevated.

Reasons to have a rest period of around 2 minutes include; you're lifting heavy and need longer to recover before the next set, you have relatively low fitness levels, and/or you are doing other training dedicated to your cardiovascular fitness.

Use 1-2 minutes of rest as a guide, and base it on the information above and how you feel at the time.

Tempo

As covered in the General Exercise Technique chapter, I recommend a 2-0-2-0 tempo or a 2-0-3-0 tempo to start with. These numbers mean that whenever the load is rising against gravity, allow 2 seconds for the movement to occur (the first 2), avoid pausing (the 0) and then take 2-3 seconds for the load to lower towards the floor, and repeat without pausing (the other 0).

This is a safe tempo because it avoids rapid, uncontrolled movements that may put unnecessary stress on the joints, muscles and connective tissue, but is also an effective tempo as the muscles have sufficient time under tension (TUT), particularly during the lowering phase when gravity can do the work for you!

Use the 2-0-2-0 tempo as your standard tempo. If, during the last few repetitions of a set, you are finding the exercise easy, slow down the phase of the exercise where the load lowers/descends to 3 seconds to create a 2-0-3-0 tempo.

Progressing

To achieve results, you need to gradually progress your strength training. Often referred to as *Progressive Resistance Training* (PRT) in research papers, it's a vital aspect of continually seeing results and achieving goals.

There are several variables that you can progress. I do not recommend progressing these all at once, but choosing the most appropriate to you and making minor changes as often as possible. Think *little and often*.

Increase Load

Initially, this is likely to be the most important variable to progress gradually. Remember, your muscles will only adapt and become stronger/bigger if you provide them with a stimulus greater than what they are used to. So if you keep lifting the same weights, you are providing the same stimulus which your body gets used to.

You are also likely to see some significant increases in strength during the first few months of training due to neuromuscular adaptations; your nervous system and muscular system adapt to become more efficient at communicating with each other to produce the necessary force, coordination and stability to carry out the exercise.

This accumulates to significant early progress. Since your strength is likely to increase, you need to respond by increasing the stimulus (the load in this case) to keep up the progress. Remember, listen to your body and progress in small increments and only as often as you feel is appropriate.

Increase Repetitions

As you get stronger, you will be able to lift the same load more times. This would be an increase in repetitions. So lifting 10kg 12 times and then a couple of weeks later lifting the same 10kg 15 times shows a progression in repetitions. Although this is a progression, it is unlikely that this is the most appropriate progression for you.

We discussed the muscular outcomes of strength training earlier, outlining the difference between muscular strength, muscular hypertrophy, and muscular endurance. We also determined that a hypertrophy rep range of 6-12, is likely to be most relevant to the goals of this over 50. So if you focus your progressions on increasing reps, you may end up well into the muscular endurance range, which may not align with your goals.

I suggest using a rep range and increasing repetitions within that rep range over several weeks. When you can comfortably achieve the highest number of reps in that range, it's time to focus on another progression rather than increasing reps more.

For example, you plan your rep range to be 10-12. You start week 1, performing 10 reps of each exercise, and by week 2 you may get to 10 and feel like you can do one more, so you continue to 11. In weeks 3-4, you are achieving a comfortable 12 reps of each exercise. The next step would be to increase the load (or another progression if more appropriate) and go back to 10 reps and repeat the process.

Increase Sets

The number of sets won't change too significantly, but it largely affects the volume of the session and, therefore, the time. I suggest 2-4 sets of each exercise, starting with 2 sets.

Sets are not a vital progression, but if you want to increase the volume of the session or you feel you aren't quite getting enough out of 2 sets, then progress to 3 and then potentially 4 in the future.

Over 3 sets are unnecessary for most people, and more than 4 is very unlikely to have any noticeable benefit to your results, and may increase your risk of injury due to fatigue.

Decrease Rest

Rest time is relevant to the training outcome. Muscular hypertrophy training, between 6-12 repetitions, requires a rest time of approximately 1-2 minutes. It's recommended to start this at the higher end, and gradually reduce it as your recovery between sets improves.

If you have just increased the weight/load on your exercises, it's a good idea to increase your rest time temporarily while you adapt to the additional weight.

Increase Complexity

Performing the same exercises for weeks and months can get a little boring over time, so progressing the exercise often by making it a bit more complex can keep things interesting and progress your training at the same time. I've provided a few exercise progressions in the 8-week plans, and you can find more variations in the bonus material.

Increase Volume & Time

If you feel you want to make your training sessions longer, you can always progress volume via the number of exercises you perform. A strength training session, including warm up and cool down, should last anywhere from 20 to 60 minutes.

Start with around 20 minutes and if you have the desire, increase to 40 minutes. If you want to increase the length of the session beyond 40 minutes, then I suggest including other components of fitness such as mobility, flexibility, balance and core. We will cover these in-depth in books 2-6 of the *Simple Fitness After 50* series.

One important point to remember when increasing the number of strength training exercises performed is program balance, particularly between pushes and pulls, as outlined earlier in this chapter. If you imbalance the program between pushes and pulls, ensure you have more pulls than pushes.

Increase Frequency

Increasing the frequency of training, how often you complete a session, is a progression. However, there becomes a point where the increased frequency can become detrimental to your results. As there are many components of fitness that are important to those over 50 (covered in the *Simple Fitness After 50* Series), I recommend starting with a strength training frequency of two sessions per week, and progressing to three sessions per week once it becomes more of a habit.

8 Week Example Programs

Below, you'll find a progressive 8-week program based on two sessions per week. I have also produced printable PDF versions which include exercise diagrams as part of the bonus material, along with the exercise technique videos.

Week 1

Session 1

Exercise	Sets	Reps	Rest
Glute Bridge	2	10-12	1.5-2 mins
Seated Band Row	2	10-12	1.5-2 mins
Kettlebell Deadlift	2	10-12	1.5-2 mins
Wall Push Ups	2	10-12	1.5-2 mins
Farmer's Walk	2	30s	1.5-2 mins

Session 2

Exercise	Sets	Reps	Rest
Chair Squats	2	10-12	1.5-2 mins
Close-Grip Pulldown	2	10-12	1.5-2 mins
Bodyweight Step Ups	2	10-12	1.5-2 mins
Dumbbell Shoulder Press	2	10-12	1.5-2 mins
Suitcase Walk	2	15s/side	1.5-2 mins

Week 2

Session 1

Exercise	Sets	Reps	Rest
Glute Bridge	2	10-12	1.5-2 mins
Seated Band Row	2	10-12	1.5-2 mins
Kettlebell Deadlift	2	10-12	1.5-2 mins
Wall Push Ups	2	10-12	1.5-2 mins
Farmer's Walk	2	30s	1.5-2 mins

Session 2

Exercise	Sets	Reps	Rest
Chair Squats	2	10-12	1.5-2 mins
Close-Grip Pulldown	2	10-12	1.5-2 mins
Bodyweight Step Ups	2	10-12	1.5-2 mins
Dumbbell Shoulder Press	2	10-12	1.5-2 mins
Suitcase Walk	2	15s/side	1.5-2 mins

Weeks 1-2

Week 3

Session 1

Exercise	Sets	Reps	Rest
Weighted Glute Bridge	2	10-12	1-2 mins
Seated One-Arm Band Row	2	10-12	1-2 mins
Kettlebell Deadlift	2	10-12	1-2 mins
Raised Push Ups	2	10-12	1-2 mins
Farmer's Walk	2	40s	1-2 mins

Session 2

Exercise	Sets	Reps	Rest
Bodyweight Squats	2	10-12	1-2 mins
Close-Grip One-Arm Pulldown	2	10-12	1-2 mins
Weighted Step Ups	2	10-12	1-2 mins
Dumbbell Shoulder Press	2	10-12	1-2 mins
Suitcase Walk	2	20s/side	1-2 mins

Week 4

Session 1

Exercise	Sets	Reps	Rest
Weighted Glute Bridge	2	10-12	1-2 mins
Seated One-Arm Band Row	2	10-12	1-2 mins
Kettlebell Deadlift	2	10-12	1-2 mins
Raised Push Ups	2	10-12	1-2 mins
Farmer's Walk	2	40s	1-2 mins

Session 2

Exercise	Sets	Reps	Rest
Bodyweight Squats	2	10-12	1-2 mins
Close-Grip One-Arm Pulldown	2	10-12	1-2 mins
Weighted Step Ups	2	10-12	1-2 mins
Dumbbell Shoulder Press	2	10-12	1-2 mins
Suitcase Walk	2	20s/side	1-2 mins

Weeks 3-4

8 WEEK PROGRAM   155

Week 5

Session 1

Exercise	Sets	Reps	Rest
Bodyweight Hip Thrusts	2	10-12	1-2 mins
Standing One-Arm Band Row	2	10-12	1-2 mins
Suitcase Deadlift	2	10-12	1-2 mins
Raised Push Ups	2	10-12	1-2 mins
Suitcase Walk	2	25s/side	1-2 mins

Session 2

Exercise	Sets	Reps	Rest
Goblet Squats	2	10-12	1-2 mins
Lat Pulldown	2	10-12	1-2 mins
Bodyweight Lateral Step Ups	2	10-12	1-2 mins
Kettlebell Overhead Press	2	10-12	1-2 mins
Rack Walk	2	20s/side	1-2 mins

Week 6

Session 1

Exercise	Sets	Reps	Rest
Bodyweight Hip Thrusts	2	10-12	1-2 mins
Standing One-Arm Band Row	2	10-12	1-2 mins
Suitcase Deadlift	2	10-12	1-2 mins
Raised Push Ups	2	10-12	1-2 mins
Farmer's Walk	2	50s	1-2 mins

Session 2

Exercise	Sets	Reps	Rest
Goblet Squats	2	10-12	1-2 mins
Lat Pulldown	2	10-12	1-2 mins
Bodyweight Lateral Step Ups	2	10-12	1-2 mins
Kettlebell Overhead Press	2	10-12	1-2 mins
Rack Walk	2	20s/side	1-2 mins

Weeks 5-6

Week 7

Session 1

Exercise	Sets	Reps	Rest
Weighted Hip Thrusts	2	10-12	1-2 mins
Single-Arm Row	2	10-12	1-2 mins
Single-Leg Deadlift	2	10-12	1-2 mins
¾ Push Ups	2	10-12	1-2 mins
Suitcase Walk	2	25s/side	1-2 mins

Session 2

Exercise	Sets	Reps	Rest
Goblet Squats	2	10-12	1-2 mins
Lat Pulldown	2	10-12	1-2 mins
Weighted Lateral Step Ups	2	10-12	1-2 mins
Kettlebell Overhead Press	2	10-12	1-2 mins
Rack Walk	2	25s/side	1-2 mins

Week 8

Session 1

Exercise	Sets	Reps	Rest
Weighted Hip Thrusts	2	10-12	1-1.5 mins
Single-Arm Row	2	10-12	1-1.5 mins
Single-Leg Deadlift	2	10-12	1-1.5 mins
¾ Push Ups	2	10-12	1-1.5 mins
Farmer's Walk	2	50s	1-1.5 mins

Session 2

Exercise	Sets	Reps	Rest
Goblet Squats	2	10-12	1-1.5 mins
Lat Pulldown	2	10-12	1-1.5 mins
Weighted Lateral Step Ups	2	10-12	1-1.5 mins
Kettlebell Overhead Press	2	10-12	1-1.5 mins
Rack Walk	2	25s/side	1-1.5 mins

Weeks 7-8

Chapter 13

Conclusion

Congratulations on completing *Fundamental Strength Training After 50*!

I hope this is just the start of your journey toward a healthier and better functioning life, and that you feel confident in what you need to focus on to make the most of your muscle-strengthening activities.

The science and research don't lie; strength training has many benefits for people of all ages, including those beyond 50. If one or more of the following benefits resonates with you, it's time to get started today...

- Improves your ability to function more effectively and efficiently in work-based environments, particularly during the last 10-15 years of your career when physical tasks become more challenging.
- Improves your ability to carry out activities of daily living with more ease and less discomfort.
- Allows you to enjoy an active role with your grandchildren.
- Helps maintain a desirable body shape and size.
- Increases resting metabolic rate, allowing you to consume more daily calories without putting on body fat.

- Reduces your risk of age-related conditions such as Type 2 Diabetes and Osteoporosis.
- Lowers the risk of fall-related injuries.

Strength training doesn't need to be complicated. Simplify it by focusing on *the essential eight* movement patterns. Use these to form the foundation of your muscle-strengthening activities and not only will you see significant results, but you're likely to do it in a safe and effective manner.

Technique is key. Study the detailed instructions for each exercise, use my exercise technique videos in the bonus material, and seek feedback from a fitness professional. You can do this in your local area, or contact me about my exercise technique analysis service where you can submit videos of your exercises and receive detailed feedback on your technique.

Once you've mastered the technique of an exercise, it's time to apply the *principle of progressive overload*! Lift a sufficient weight that causes you to reach the point of fatigue at the end of each set. To maximize results, it should be a challenge to finish your last few repetitions of each set.

Use my 8-week program to get you started TODAY. If you prefer to use a printable PDF version with diagrams of the exercises included, access the bonus material to receive them for FREE.

Remember that a multi-component approach to fitness will provide the best outcome for a fit and healthy future. Check out the rest of the *Simple Fitness After 50* series and subscribe for updates and book release notifications by visiting mikewilsonfitness.com

If you want to take things to another level and continue your fitness journey through any of my coaching services, check out www.lifetimefitnesscoaching.com

Thank You and Please!

Thank you so much for taking the time to read **Fundamental Strength Training After 50**. I'm truly grateful to you all and hope that you found it to be informative and helpful towards your health & fitness goals.

If you enjoyed this book, please consider letting other people know by leaving a review on Amazon.

Amazon reviews are incredibly helpful; both for self-published authors like myself to get the word out, and also for other potential readers to decide whether this book will be useful to them. Thank you in advance. I'm truly grateful for your support.

To leave a review, please return to the product page on Amazon, scroll down to the review section and click the "Write a customer review" button.

To find the product page on Amazon, either search "Fundamental Strength Training After 50" or "B0B1Z7443J", or scan the QR code on the following page using your phone camera.

Amazon US Reviews

Amazon UK Reviews

Thanks again!

Mike

Author Bio

Mike is a 1:1 Online Fitness Coach, Fitness Educator and Author living in the UK.

Mike obtained a degree in Sport & Exercise Science at University and has since spent over 20 years in the fitness industry. He currently runs Lifetime Fitness Coaching, The Fitness Education Hub, as well as writing and teaching fitness industry qualifications in Spain and Malta. More recently, Mike has also become a self-published fitness author.

Mike currently specialises in three main areas:

1) Coaching and educating adults over 50 years of age to lose weight, maximize their health & fitness, increase their functional capabilities in daily activities and sports, and reduce their risk of future health problems associated with a sedentary lifestyle.

2) Educating future fitness professionals to obtain their Gym Instructor, Personal Trainer, and CPD qualifications with the - European Personal Training Institute, at their campuses in Spain and Malta. Mike has been tutoring and assessing fitness qualifications for over 15 years and prides himself on explaining complex subjects in a logical, easy to understand, and fun way.

3) His latest venture focuses more on online entrepreneurship within the fitness industry. Working on multiple online revenue streams and passing this knowledge on to current Fitness

Professionals to enhance *their* online revenue streams. This includes areas such as self-publishing books, online course creation, online fitness coaching, email marketing, blogging, and eCommerce.

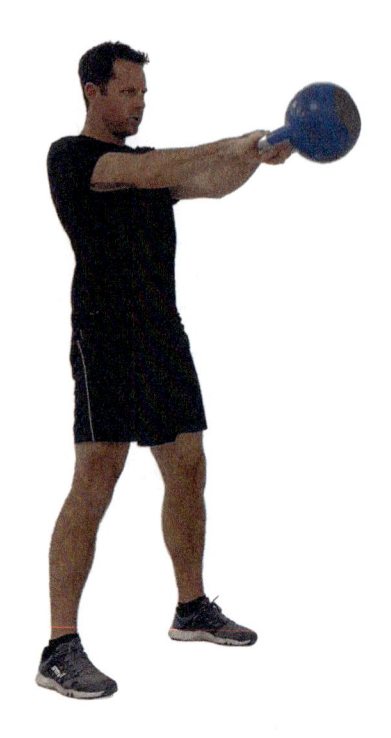

Mike Wilson

Coming Soon

Fundamental Strength Training After 50 is book one of the *Simple Fitness After 50* series. The series covers the fundamental components of fitness for those over 50 years of age. Go to mikewilsonfitness.com to register for updates on upcoming releases.

The aim of the book series is to simplify what exercises are important to improve all 5 components of fitness; to maintain freedom & independence in later life, improve body composition, be able to perform activities of daily living with more ease, decrease the risk of age-related diseases, and live life with more energy and vitality.

The remaining four books in the series are:

Fundamental Core Training After 50 (Book Two)

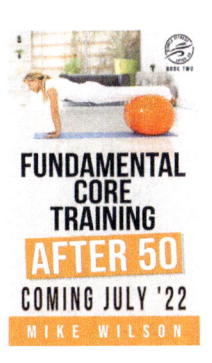

Fundamental Balance Training After 50 (Book Three)

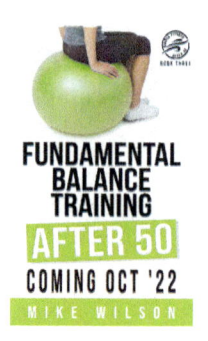

Fundamental Flexibility & Mobility After 50 (Book Four)

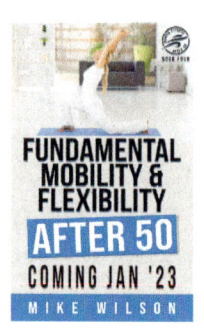

Fundamental Posture Training After 50 (Book Five)

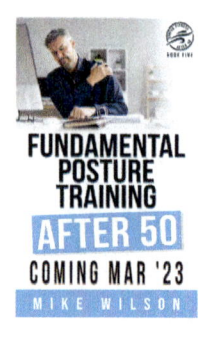

Bibliography

American College of Sports Medicine. (2010). ACSM's Guidelines for Exercise Testing and Prescription. Eighth Edition. *Philadelphia: Wolters Kluwer/Lippincott Williams & Wilkins.*

Butler-Browne, G., et. al. (2018). How Muscles Age, and How Exercise Can Slow It. *The Scientist.*

Centers for Disease Control and Prevention. "Keep on Your Feet - Preventing Older Adult Falls." Accessed January, 2022. CDC.gov/injury/features/older-adult-falls/index.html

Chodzko-Zajko, W.J. (2014). ACSM's exercise for older adults. *Philadelphia: Wolters Kluwer/Lippincott Williams & Wilkins.*

DiPietro, L. (2019). Physical Activity and Function in Older Age: It's Never too Late to Start! *American College of Sports Medicine.* Accessed May, 2022. https://www.acsm.org/blog-detail/acsm-blog/2019/09/10/physical-activity-function-older-age

Griffin, R.M. (2021). Myths About Exercise and Older Adults. *Compass by WebMD.* Accessed January, 2022. https://www.webmd.com/healthy-aging/features/exercise-older-adults#1

Harvard Health Publishing. (2016). Preserve your muscle mass. Accessed January, 2022. https://www.health.harvard.edu/staying-healthy/preserve-your-muscle-mass/

Hong, A.R., & Kim, S.W. (2018). Effects of Resistance Exercise on Bone Health. *Endocrinology and Metabolism (Seoul, Korea), 33 (4), 435–444.* https://doi.org/10.3803/EnM.2018.33.4.435

Liu, C. J., & Latham, N. K. (2009). Progressive resistance strength training for improving physical function in older adults. *The Cochrane database of systematic reviews*, *2009*(3), CD002759. https://doi.org/10.1002/14651858.CD002759.pub2

Seguin, R.A., et.al. (2002) Growing Stronger: Strength Training for Older Adults. *Division of Nutrition and Physical Activity.*

The Physical Activity Readiness Questionnaire for Everyone (PAR-Q+). https://eparmedx.com/?page_id=75

World Health Organization (2008). WHO global report on falls prevention in older age. *Geneva: World Health Organization.*

World Health Organization (2020). WHO guidelines on physical activity and sedentary behaviour. *Geneva: World Health Organization.*

Printed in Great Britain
by Amazon